TISSUE LEVEL HYPOGLYCEMIA

A NOVEL MECHANISM OF TISSUE DAMAGE DURING SHOCK IN NEWBORNS

Dr. ALOKE V.R

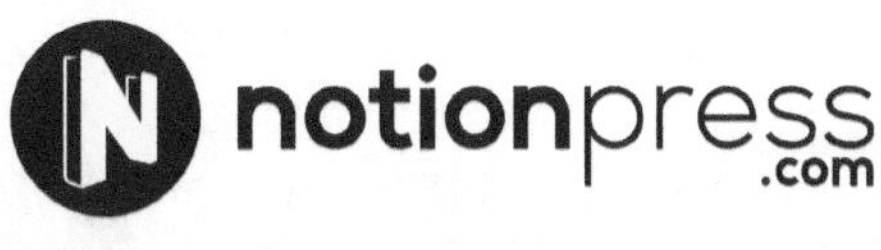

ISBN 979-8-89186-384-2

DEDICATION

This book is dedicated to all my babies who silently taught me the concept of Tissue Level Hypoglycemia.

Contents

Preface

Medical fraternity is a rapidly progressing field especially during the last 2 decades. In the field of Neonatology more and more under 1000 gm babies are surviving with and without morbidity. Even after years of technological progress we are not able to send babies out of NICU without morbidity. Mortality is also a common occurrence. Moreover, we are not able to mimic the environment and conditions of a human womb in comfort and outcome. Why are we losing so many babies to mortality and morbidity? Why is this happening? A simple explanation is that we have not fully mastered the mechanisms of human physiology and processes involved in brain damage. Frankly speaking we have not yet mastered the complexities of the human body. But we have the false pride of knowing everything, it may take one or two centuries before we master at least something. For making faster progress in understanding the complexities of the human body we have to challenge and question the existing theories and put forward new ones. There is a great inertia (resistance) in the scientific community towards drastic changes. Artificial barriers are kept to prevent rapid changes, whether these barriers are for good or bad only time will tell.

During my 20 years of neonatal practice there were several situations where we were not able to explain the reasons for the development delay or the neurological abnormalities even after giving good neonatal care and without obvious insult to the baby. *Neurology of newborns* by Volpe has tried its best to explain things in prospective but still in many areas it has failed to explain fully. Out of curiosity and to find a rational explanation for things I myself conceptualized several hypotheses. In this book I am describing one of the most promising hypotheses that is, **"Tissue level hypoglycemia during shock"**, the silent master assassin in tissue damage during shock.

Currently no scientific community ever accepts concepts based on hearsay. Strong evidences are required for every hypothesis. For implementing new therapeutic modality strong backup of evidence-based medicine is required. Then comes the question has evidence-based medicine hindered the progress of entry of breakthrough concepts. My personal answer is yes. Majority of our evidences are from RCT's and meta-analysis. Can we prove everything based on human studies, no we cannot, there are several limitations and hurdles doing human studies. Once a new idea comes to our mind it should evolve into a hypothesis and then one has to prove that hypothesis though studies, but human studies have their own limitations. This limitation can be grouped into two categories, one is the difficulty in doing human studies and second is its limitation in interpretation biases. In my opinion there should be balance between Evidence-based medicine and Practice-based evidence. We doctors are not thinking beyond our self-made boundaries. The reason being that nobody hears your theories without evidence, nobody is willing for a theoretical discussion, there are no platforms for youngsters to expressing their theories. Proving theories through studies are not easy for majority of practicing doctors, simple concepts can be proved easily through studies. But if your concept is more complex then you reach a dead end.

In the current scenario a concept or hypothesis will be summarily rejected without solid proof. Some degree of theoretical discussions should be encouraged by the elite scientific community only then will new ideas and concepts will come.

I am doing critical care practice in neonatology and Pediatrics for the last 20 years. Through this book I am putting forward some of my explanations and hypothesis for some of the unexplained outcomes in these fields. Bringing out these ideas through my second book as journal publications are out of reach for the ordinary without evidence! These are huge limitations for RCT and other studies when your theories are at the molecular level. There are limitations for studies for the majority of doctors and we should know our limitations. **Limitations in studies should not limit our ability to produce new concepts for the unexplained.**

This book is entirely different in that only those with an open mind to new ideas and concepts should go through it. My aim is to spread new concepts critically analyze it, reject it, accept it or build over it and bring useful changes for the patients. Albert Einstein's *General theory of relativity* took years to get approved and accepted, still people are searching in the darkness. When you reach a dead end in explaining things, your only tool is your brain and use of thought experiments for developing new hypotheses. That is what I have done and arrived at a self-convincing conclusion. Converting these into studies for finding the truth is beyond my capability (but trying) so I am expressing my views through a book for a wider discussion. My first book named *"Practicing without Evidence"* for practicing Neonatologist and Pediatrician had mentioned these theories. One of the most promising concepts in that book is the tissue level hypoglycemia occurring during shock and I am discussing that in this book in detail. I request all readers to dig deeper into the concept and critically analyze and arrive at your own conclusions.

Birth is a real testing time for all babies especially preterm babies. They are leaving the comfort of womb and venturing outside to lead an independent life. Damage to developing organs especially brain can occur during birth or after that, infections are an additional insult waiting to happen. There are multiple factors all leading finally to damage individual neurons. Insults can be hypoglycemia, hypoxia, shock, infections, intracranial hemorrhages of varied variety and sizes, electrolyte imbalance related, seizure to name a handful. Most of these are gross thing happening to the brain and what happens at the microscopic level to produce tissue damage is really unknown or minimally known. If we know the mechanisms well, we can develop therapies to lessen its impact. If you analyze hypoglycemia causing brain damage, we don't know the exact molecular pathways to the damage. For example, some babies with a blood sugar value of 50 mg/ dl can produce seizure and brain damage. Another baby with a blood sugar value of 35 mg/dl can be perfectly normal and found accidently during routine screening. We don't know whether the absolute value of blood sugar is the actual culprit or some other factors which is co damaging the brain. Only if we know all the mechanisms occurring inside the cell at molecular level, we can say with cent percent conviction that the damage is due to this or that. We humans are not yet reached that stage. This is the case with GM hemorrhage, several theories are floating, but why there is bleed at that place and why there is an increased vulnerability during those early days, we can grossly say that, it is due to some hemodynamic instability, these are just assumptions and not a convincing molecular level conclusion. Proving each theory is not that easy. But we should keep on trying and on the way some promising theories may prop up. Promising theories should face wider discussions and research.

From my experience over the years, I have observed that shock in its mildest form (subtle or subclinical shock) is missed by many doctors or is given less importance and this monster is wrecking silent havoc in tissue damage. So, I tried to over treat shock and to my surprise we started seeing less and less brain damage, less neonatal seizures, less apnea, faster recoveries, less and less higher degrees of GM-IVH. Digging deeper into this I found several new things to my surprise.

It is through the circulation that the external world (through oxygen) is in constant contact with all the cells of the body. We are supplying each cell with oxygen, glucose, all the mineral and micronutrients required through the medium of blood called perfusion. We are also removing waste molecules from them. Any minor fault in this can affect individual cell. The requirements of cells also varies and so also resistant to lack of supply. Neurons are the one with stringent supply norms and any compromise will manifest immediately.

Analyzing the nutrient supply to individual cells in normal state and during shock I came across one amazing discovery of the role played by glucose. Glucose is in dynamic equilibrium balancing supply and demand and during shock there is supply disruption of glucose and results in tissue level hypoglycemia, which is masked by the blood normoglycemia. This I call "tissue level hypoglycemia occurring during shock". The mechanisms are explained in the subsequent chapters. The tissue level hypoglycemia is hidden and never comes into the open picture. There are no surrogate markers at present for the tissue level hypoglycemia. Tissues are damaged due to the inadequate supply of glucose during shock, which is the real destroyer of tissues. During shock this cellular level hypoglycemia is never discussed anywhere. This is the topic of discussion of this book. For clearer view shock needs to be discussed in detail slightly different from the conventional views.

– Dr. Aloke V.R
MD, DCH, DM (Neo)
Consultant Neonatologist
Nyle Hospital, Thrissur, Kerala

Chapter-1

Physiology of Tissue level Micro-circulation during Shock and Normal – A Different Perspective (Oxygen-Glucose Dyad)

This chapter is to lay a common foundation for the reader so that a wider discussion is possible. We are from different backgrounds and so a direct discussion on the topic can lead to misunderstanding. Most important thing in this book is shock and we have to arrive at a common platform before we start analyzing it.

Everybody is well aware of the normal tissue circulation and its regulations and I will be discussing this from a different perspective. This discussion is to bring the reader and writer onto a same platform so that we see the same thing at the microscopic level. This minute scrutiny will help us in understanding the concept of "Tissue level Hypoglycemia" (discussed in the subsequent chapters) the main hidden culprit in brain damage.

Normal oxygen transport – What is exactly happening?

At the alveolar end

Oxygen reaching the alveoli rapidly dissolves into the interstitial fluid surrounding the alveoli which then gets into the capillary plasma and from there into RBC plasma and finally get attached to the RBC hemoglobin in a cooperative kinetic manner. This means that there is no direct transport of oxygen from alveoli into the RBC hemoglobin and whatever FiO2 reaching the alveoli has to first get dissolve in the interstitial fluid then into plasma and finally get attached to the hemoglobin. This creates a limitation in the oxygen transport through the blood (this may be the protective strategy against oxygen toxicity). Oxygen has very low solubility in plasma and interstitial fluid and the relationship is **linearly** related. The coefficient for dissolved oxygen transport is 0.0031ml oxygen per mm Hg O2/dL (1) The amount of oxygen transported by 100ml of plasma in dissolved form at 100 mm Hg of partial pressure in the alveoli is

= 100 x 0.0031 ml = 0.3 ml of oxygen/dL (room air FIO2 =21%)

- **Amount of O2 transported through 15g of hemoglobin is 19.5 ml of O2/dL at a FIO2 of 21%,**
- **Amount of O2 transported in dissolved form is just 0.3 ml/dl**
- **Hb bound O2 vs Dissolved O2 = 19.5ml vs 0.3ml, 98.5% vs 1.5%**

This 0.3ml Oxygen/dl increases to 2.1 ml of oxygen/dL when FIO2 reaches 100% (700 x 0.0031 = 2.1 ml/dL)

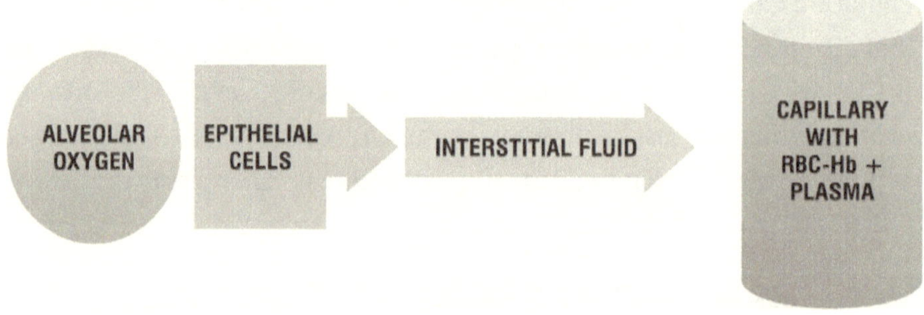

Figure: 1.1: Transport of oxygen from alveoli into RBC

Major portion of oxygen is transported through hemoglobin (98.5%) under room air condition and this decreases to 90% when FiO2 is increased to 100%, the rest 10% is transported in dissolved form. This shows that oxygen carried through blood (hemoglobin (RBC) and plasma) is limited by the amount of hemoglobin concentration present. Oxygen transport from alveoli to tissues can be compared to shuttle bus transport system.

Two types of transport can occur in a bus, as seated and standing, seated form corresponds to oxygen carried by hemoglobin and standing corresponds to dissolved oxygen transport. In seated form the amount of oxygen transported is limited by the number of seats available or the number of molecules of hemoglobin available. In the standing position the transportable numbers are variable, either you can run jam packed or run loosely packed, this depends on the number of passengers eager to get into the bus (corresponding to the FiO2 concentration) at the bus stop. In bus stop there are only standing people which corresponds to the dissolved oxygen and this capacity is limited. But high turnover is possible provided the bus arrives (Hb) arrives more frequently (if blood circulates fast with higher Hb concentration). This oxygen transport from alveoli to hemoglobin in RBC is rapid and it takes only 0.1 second and it happens during one third length of transit through alveolar capillaries (fig: 1.1 &1.2). The distance between the air within the alveoli and the blood in the capillaries is approximately 0.7 microns (700nm). This distance is 2300 times the diameter of the oxygen molecule (oxygen molecule diameter is 0.3 nm) (1 micron =1000 nm) and 700 times the diameter of glucose molecule (glucose molecule diameter is 1 nm). If we imagine us (25 cm diameter) in the place of oxygen molecule we have to walk 0.5 km (0.25 m x 2300 =575 meters) before we reach capillary blood from alveoli. This applies to tissue end capillaries also.

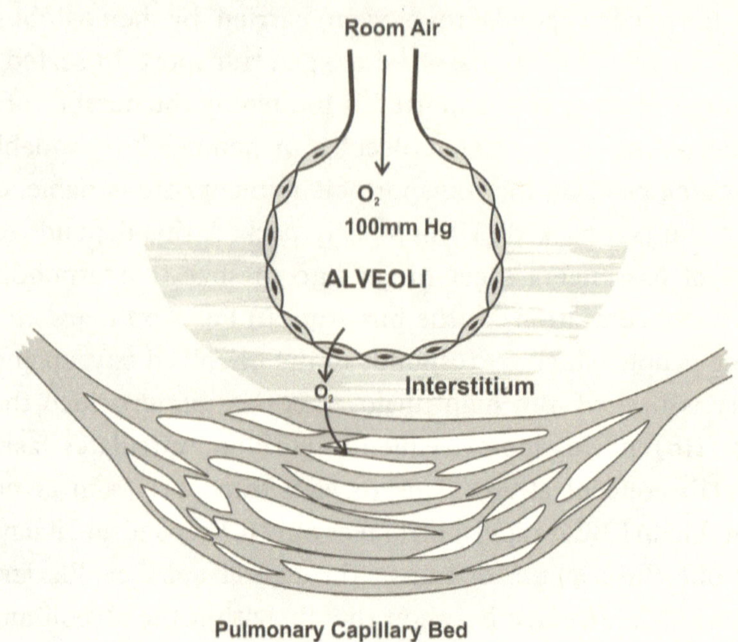

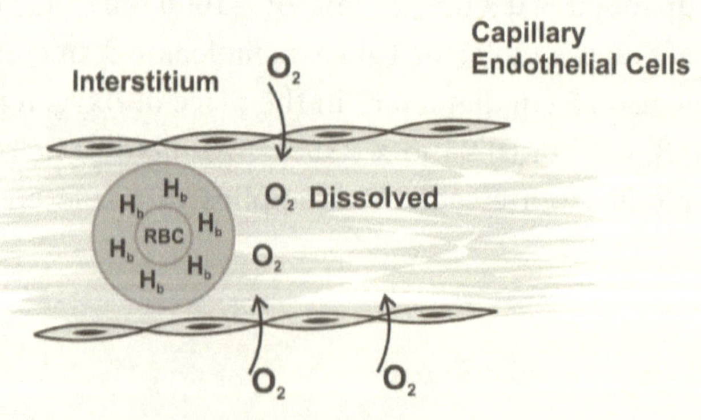

Figure: 1.2: Oxygen transport from alveoli to capillary blood.

Summary of oxygen transported from alveoli

- Oxygen carried bound to hemoglobin (major)
- Oxygen dissolved in RBC cytoplasm (negligible)
- Oxygen dissolved in plasma (minimal)

Table: 1.1: Amount of Oxygen transported (1)

Alveolar FIO2 = 21%	Alveolar FIO2 = 100%	Difference (%)
O2 carried binding to Hb = 19.5ml (98.5%)	O2 carried binding to Hb = 19.5ml (90%)	Nil (0%)
O2 dissolved in plasma = 0.3 ml (1.5%)	O2 dissolved in plasma = 2.1 ml (10%)	**1.8 ml (8.5%)**
O2 dissolved in RBC water = negligible	O2 dissolved in RBC water = negligible	Nil
Total O2 carried = 19.8 ml (100%)	Total O2 carried = 21.6 ml (100%)	**1.8 ml**
Increasing FIO2 from 21% to 100% causes increase of only 1.8ml (8.5%) of additional oxygen transport through 100 ml of blood. Hemoglobin is the real determinant of amount of oxygen transported.		

At the tissue End

As this plasma oxygen and oxygen bound to hemoglobin moves forward it mixes with blood from other areas and reaches heart and is distributed to all areas, the dissolved oxygen content and hemoglobin bound oxygen will be same till arterioles and capillary bed. Once capillary bed is reached oxygen diffuses into the interstitial fluid which is continuously and rapidly taken up by the cells. The RBC cannot pass into the interstitial fluid and capillary plasma oxygen is in dynamic equilibrium with the interstitial fluid oxygen. RBC bound oxygen cannot be directly transferred into the interstitial fluid or directly into the cells. RBC is continuously supplying oxygen to the capillary plasma and which in turn is supplying it to the interstitial fluid from where cells can take oxygen. During this transfer there is no medium which can acts as a reserve for oxygen. Only the continuous flow of RBC can act as a reservoir of oxygen. So, whenever this flow of capillary RBC slows (as in early stages of shock) it effects cellular oxygen supply instantaneously. Shock effects the tissue oxygen supply immediately and those with high metabolic rate will be affected most i.e., the neurons.

RBC – Hb bound oxygen + plasma dissolved oxygen → interstitial dissolved oxygen → cells

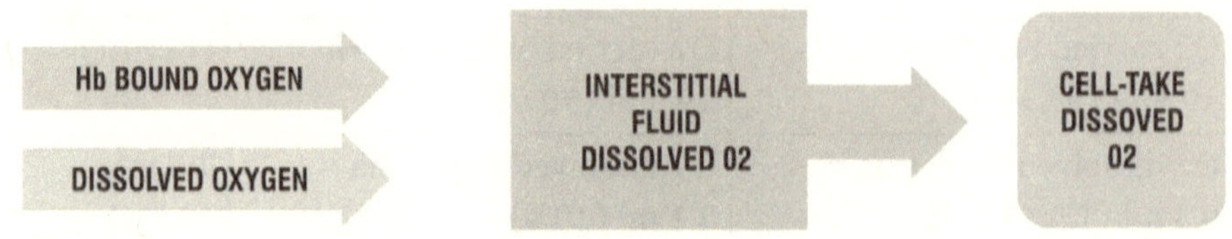

Figure: 1.3: Oxygen transport at the Capillary End

Important points:

- Alveolar oxygen cannot directly attach to hemoglobin, first it has to dissolve in interstitial fluid and then enter RBC. Even though the distance is small there is a space barrier.

- Alveolar oxygen and dissolved interstitial fluid oxygen concentration is linearly related. Moreover, the solubility of oxygen in this fluid is very less. Molecular motion propels oxygen through interstitial fluid into RBC and then attaches to hemoglobin.

- Similarly, hemoglobin bound oxygen cannot directly supply oxygen to the tissues

- Hemoglobin bound oxygen just act as a carrier, supplying O2 continuously to maintain plasma oxygen tension and interstitial fluid oxygen tension at the tissue end.

- Plasma dissolved oxygen and interstitial dissolved oxygen are in a continuous dynamic equilibrium

- From dissolved oxygen in the interstitial fluid cells take up oxygen continuously.

- **As long as capillary perfusion is good, interstitial dissolved oxygen content will be maintained and cells requirements are met. This is a dynamic equilibrium state (there is continuous supply and continuous uptake, and no reservoir) and the cells are affected the moment supply is compromised (as in shock).**

What happens during shock?

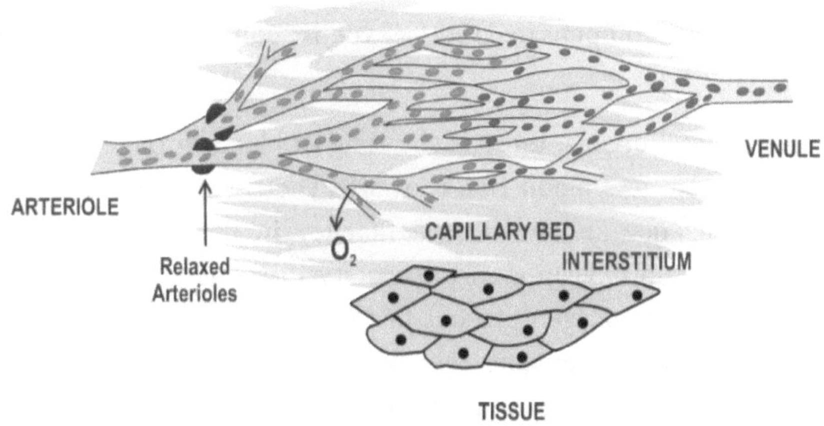

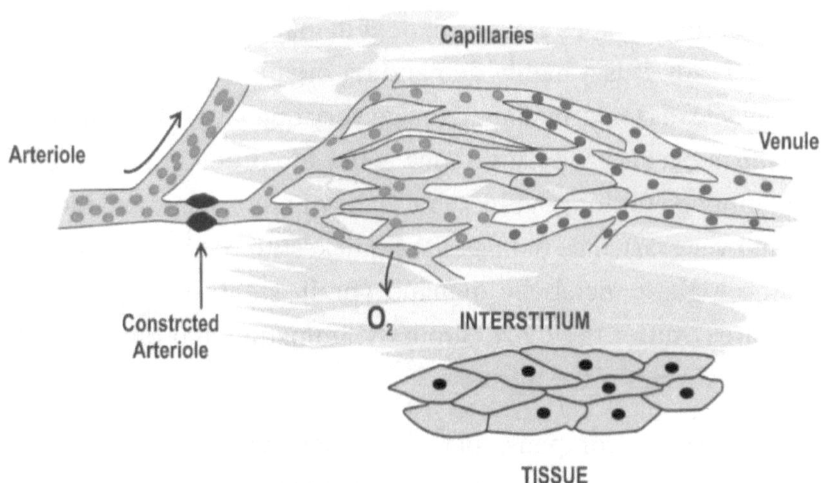

Figure: 1.4: Capillary Circulation during Normal state and in Shock

Simple definition of shock is: **when circulation is unable to meet the tissue requirements of oxygen and nutrients.** During shock the preference of body changes. Body wants to save the vital organs at the expense of the non-vital organs, so body shunts blood away from non-vital organs (skin, GIT, muscles) to vital organs (brain, heart, kidneys). In the vital organs for example the brain, there are preferential allotments to vital centers (brain stem, basal ganglia, grey matter areas are compensated) at the expense of non-vital areas (white matter) (fig: 1.4).

In the non-vital organs, there is shunting of blood through arteriolar constriction, so less blood flows towards the tissues, this creates an oxygen deficiency and nutrient deficiency in the interstitial fluid. Since there is no oxygen storage capacity in the interstitial fluid, in no time whatever oxygen present in the interstitial fluid is used up. It is a dynamic instantaneous deficiency and cells shift to anaerobic metabolism. Most of the non-vital organs (skin, GIT) are resistant towards hypoxia for long periods unless supply restrictions are very severe. Muscles and skin are highly resistant to hypoxic damage and they can vary greatly their metabolic requirements. These organs due to their flexibility escapes any permanent damage. But this is not the case with the brain, it is a highly demanding organ and significant oxygen deficiency leads to permanent damage very quickly. The compensatory mechanism occurring during shock is not foolproof and is not perfect. So, it cannot go for long. Vulnerable areas of brain, heart and kidney get damaged very fast. The damages are quickest to the brain. Those areas with the highest metabolic demand (brain stem, basal ganglia, grey matter area) suffer the most. Similarly, immature and rapidly growing areas of brain suffer the most.

During subtle or compensatory shock, less vital areas of the brain, like periventricular white matter suffers the most. In these cases, vital areas will be perfused at the expense of periventricular areas and it suffers mildly but for a prolonged period. Clinically severe shock will be tackled quickly or otherwise the baby will die. But subtle shock can remain undetected for extended periods under a less trained eye. These produce small damages but for extended periods producing cystic PVL, microcephaly etc. on MRI scan. In severe shock any area of the brain can get affected.

During shock, areas of brain affected can be divided into

- Compensated areas or vital brain areas (vital for survival) like brain stem, basal ganglia, grey matter etc.
- Non-compensated areas or less vital areas like periventricular white matter and other white matter areas.

Compensated areas are relatively protected at the expense of less vital areas. This temporary adjustment cannot last long as in long run all areas will be affected. During shock body's priority is immediate survival rather that prevention of long-term neurological deficit. But we treating doctors should be concerned about both, immediate survival as well as long-term consequences.

My idea of discussion is to bring forth the importance of subtle shock (subclinical shock) in producing brain damage. Shock is described in detail in my own language in subsequent chapters. The moment the baby goes into shock there are areas which are compromised but measuring the degree of compromise and damage is difficult. In the case of newborn premature brain, the areas affected are the periventricular white matter and other white matter areas, rapidly growing and multiplying germinal matrix (GM) areas, resulting in Peri Ventricular Leukomalacia (PVL), GM-IVH. As a neonatologist we all know the burden of PVL, GM-IVH, cognitive and other deficits in the community. Are they all due to the undetected subtle shock we have missed? The answer is we don't know. We don't have a definite answer for lots of things. If at least some of them are due to the missed subtle shock, then we can prevent some of them in the future. My experience has taught me to over-treat shock rather that to under-treat it as our parameters helping in detection of subtle shock is poor. Our shock detection based on NIBP fall has very low sensitivity. Only 3 out of 10 babies (30%) will show a BP fall when there is shock, (clinical experience) others will have prolonged CRT, poor appearance of baby, weak peripheral pulsations, tachycardia, decreased urine output, altered sensorium, lethargy, seizures, apnea, development of metabolic acidosis in ABG or VBG etc. From my experience the most useful and confirmatory one out of these is the development of metabolic acidosis in the VBG/ABG. So, all sick new admissions to the NICU must have a VBG or an ABG done.

The brain is a very complex network of neurons and each neuron is precious. The preservation of each one these should be our priority. Our problem is we simplify things too much and take everything for granted. There are billions and billions of neurons with its supporting cells in the brain, we cannot make sure that all cells are well nourished in a compensated or subtle shock situation especially when it is prolonged. Shock in any form need to be treated well, over treatment will not harm the baby. We have to lower our threshold for the detection of subtle shock. If the skin color of the baby is bad or not appropriate or CRT is prolonged or if there is a development of mild metabolic acidosis it means that somewhere body is compromised. These areas are the non-vital areas, including non-vital areas of brain. As a doctor you know the long-term consequences of damage to a non-vital area like the peri ventricular white matter. For the baby all areas are vital. Prolonged compromise (even mild) to any area can produce irreparable damage. There should be no compromise towards shock. Lactate level should never be allowed to raise above normal. Base deficit (-4, − 8, − 12, − 16 mmol/L etc.) and blood lactate values are all in a dynamic equilibrium state of continuous production and removal (consumption) from body. For example, an increased lactate value of 2.5 mmol/L indicates there is anaerobic metabolism happening somewhere in the body and that there is an increased production of lactate. Simultaneously there is consumption of lactate by muscles and other tissues and a new equilibrium is reached. Only when the production of lactate is increased, new higher value of blood lactate is reached and that occurs when shock is worsened. This is the case with base deficit also. So, our aim should be to keep all these in the normal range by treating shock and its primary cause appropriately. These can be taken as surrogate markers of shock. When the lactic acid production increases the base deficit increases, kidneys and lungs are continuously working to compensate its adverse effects. That is why I called this state a dynamic equilibrium state. Increased lactic acid production means somewhere in the body anaerobic metabolism is occurring.

When you are treating a sick newborn, you should feel like a neuron and feel its suffering when compromised. Our problem is we are happy with some gross values like NIBP, HR, RR, SPO2 etc., but we should think beyond these values and get to the root cause of the problem at a microscopic level. The next section will explain why I am so obsessed with shock, the core concept of "tissue level hypoglycemia" during shock.

Normal Glucose transport and its compromise during shock.

Glucose is the substrate on which oxygen acts to release energy. Oxygen and glucose should both be readily available for smooth functioning of a cell so, both can be called as an **Oxygen-Glucose Dyad**. One is useless when other is not available. Blood plasma carries glucose to the tissues and glucose diffuses into the interstitial fluid from where cells take it. Problem happens when there is shock. During shock, circulation slows or there is blood diversion to vital organs, correspondingly, less plasma glucose reaches interstitial fluid and thus less glucose is available for the cells. Cells experience tissue level hypoglycemia; this is never highlighted anywhere. This gets exaggerated several times when there is simultaneous oxygen deficiency. During shock there is associated deficiency of oxygen and cells convert to anaerobic metabolism (anaerobic glycolysis) which is **highly inefficient** and so the requirement of glucose sky rockets. Anaerobic glycolysis is approximately **16 times** less efficient than aerobic metabolism in producing ATP, so in theory cells need 16 times more glucose to produce the same amount of ATP (aerobic – 2 ATP Vs 32 ATP anaerobic) (2, 17). [Anaerobic glycolysis is 100 times faster than oxidative phosphorylation (3)]. In non-vital organs (skin, muscles at rest) this may not be a major problem, but this can be a problem in heart, brain and kidneys. In the brain, the non-vital areas like brain white matter, periventricular areas suffer "silently" from deficiency of glucose and also oxygen. Till now this deficiency of glucose has never been highlighted, only role of oxygen deficiency is discussed. Glucose deficiency is discussed only in the contest of blood hypoglycemia. I am bringing this concept of **"tissue level hypoglycemia"** occurring **silently** during shock at cellular level into the discussion.

So, during shock along with hypoxemia to the cells there is also deficient supply of substrate glucose (both oxygen and glucose don't have a reservoir in plasma or interstitial fluid, it is a dynamic supply and consumption state, deficiency manifests instantaneously). The deficiency for glucose is more exaggerated when the cells shift to anaerobic metabolism due to its inefficiency.

The word *silent* is special because there are no surrogate markers for this **tissue level hypoglycemia**, so mostly it never gets noticed. There are only subtle signs which too are non-specific to tissue hypoglycemia and so usually get attributed to shock. If you check the blood glucose it will be normal but at tissue level there is glucose deficiency due to poor circulation. Subtle signs of tissue level glucose deficiency or tissue level poor circulation are irritability, apnea, drowsiness, seizures, tissue damage manifested as PVL changes etc. We have to try to find a surrogate marker for tissue level hypoglycemia occurring silently during shock. Till we get a clearer picture and a surrogate marker we have to consider tissue level hypoglycemia occurring along with shock. So, try to maintain higher blood glucose levels whenever these is shock. This is like giving extra oxygen during shock even if the SPO2 are in the normal range. This may be the reason for the better outcome of babies observed during HIE associated with hyperglycemia in some studies (4).

I have made a more detailed discussion on tissue level hypoglycemia in subsequent chapters. This association of silent hypoglycemia accompanying shock is never mentioned anywhere and this seems to be a new concept having longstanding consequences. This may be the missing link related to several of developmental delays seen in preterm or sick babies. If this hypothesis turns out to be correct then subtle shock and shock need to be taken more seriously and the rush to stop inotropes should not be there. Cutoff value for sugar will be upgraded to higher levels during shock and children will get better neurodevelopmental outcomes.

Currently there are so many acquired neurodevelopmental deficits like PVL, GMH, IVH, acquired microcephaly, marked cystic encephalomalacia etc. occurring in a sick preterm child which are not properly explainable with the current understanding. If there is prematurity everything is dumped on the prematurity and if the child had undergone ventilation, then that takes up all the burden. That is not the proper way of explaining things, there should be a molecular level of explanation. Let this shed light in this area and initiate a larger debate.

Chapter-2

CNS Microcirculation, Subtle Shock and Brain Damage (GM-IVH, PVL, Acquired Microcephaly)

Whenever a problem happens to a newborn premature baby, our first concern is whether there will be long term neurological consequences. Nobody is sure about the outcome and that is why everybody is worried. Let us discuss some practical aspects of brain circulation and metabolism which can shed some light into this worry. Brain is a complex organ controlling all other body parts and is composed of billions and billions of neurons and several times more supporting cells. Each neuron has 1000's of synaptic connections and these connections are the data exchange points. The ultimate performance of brain depends on the preservation of all these cells and synapses. Synaptic destruction, neuronal destruction, supporting cell destruction all will have long term neurologic consequences. Supporting cells are important in myelination, nutrition and overall health of the neurons. If the damage is happening during the early stage of development (preterm period) it is in a logarithmic proportion. Destruction of each progenitor cell or neuron in the early stage of development results in virtual destruction of 1000's of daughter cells (subsequent generations of cells). It has a cascading effect. This is similar to how the destruction of a small limb bud during the first trimester can result in the loss of entire limb.

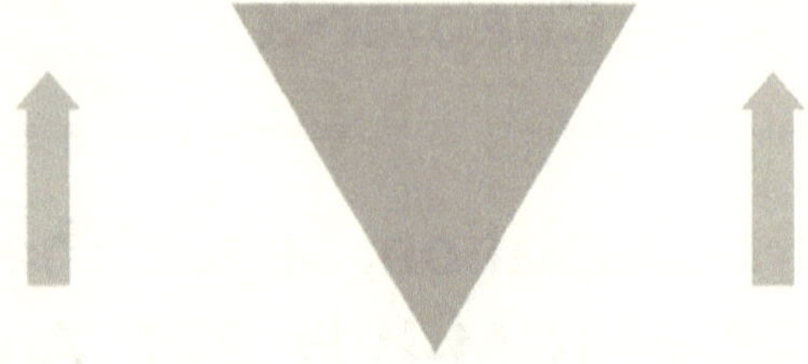

Figure: 2.1: Schematic Representation of Single cell Destruction resulting in Multiplier effect

Fetus develops from a single celled ovum and multiplies exponentially. Early damage to the fetus (in the 1st trimester) will be incompatible with life so end in miscarriages. First trimester damage result in severe organ damage as these organs are in its early development phase. Second trimester damage is also life threatening as organs are still forming. Third trimester damages are less severe.

Damages can occur in 4 ways in brain.

1. **Like destroying the bud of a sapling (during early developing stage)**

   Damage can occur to the cells destined to play a major role in future, like the cells destined for migration from germinal matrix to cerebral cortex. Damage here is deadly as a whole family of daughter neurons will be destroyed.

2. **Like destroying the formed branches of a tree (after maturation is near complete)**

   Damage can occur in the neurons in its final resting place like that occurring in the grey matter areas of cortex etc. This is less damaging compared to the first variety unless extensive.

3. **Damage can occur in a localized areas** like that occurring due to a hemorrhage into a localized area, or due to a tumor growth.

4. **Damage can occur to the whole area of brain (or body)** as occurring due to shock, hypoxemia, hypoglycemia, generalized brain oedema, asphyxia etc. In this whole brain can get affected (every cell) but intensity of involvement varies depending on the regional factors and on the intensity of insult.

After full term birth neuronal multiplication and cell migration, myelination etc. will be continuing till the age of 3 years. By 3 years 95% of the growth of brain will be over. Postnatally 70% of neuronal growth and multiplication occurs in the first 7 months of age and 90% of growth will be over by 2 years of age and rest during the 3rd year. Any insult or deficiency during this period can have varying degrees of long-term consequences. Damages during these periods is less severe compared to any damages that can occur in the fetal stage. So, practically speaking we have to be very careful when handling a preterm baby, less the maturity, more the depth of damage for the same insult.

- When caring preterm babies, be careful of the following,

    o   Not to disturb or stop the normal sequence of brain growth (neuronal proliferation, migration, organization, and myelination). Allow normal undisturbed normal growth.
    o   Not to destroy rapidly multiplying areas of brain like germinal matrix. This is possible by taking preventive measures for GM-IVH.
    o   Not to damage already formed areas like cerebral cortex, brain stem, deep nuclear areas.

Plasticity of brain (5,6,7,8)

Newborn brain development is a continuous construction and remodeling process. During brain development millions and millions of extra neurons, synapses and supporting cells are produced which are subsequently destined for destruction like a remodeling process. This cell death and elimination of neuronal processes and synapses occur during the organizational period of development. These regressive events like neuronal destruction can be modified when the brain is injured and that neurons and synapses which are destined for elimination can be retained and preserved of its function. These neurons can take over the functions of the destroyed area. In addition, new projections can develop in response to injury during this organizational period of development. This process of retaining or preserving neurons and synapses is called plasticity of brain. The same thing is seen in infants and children with neonatal stroke where the unaffected side takes over the function of the affected side at least partially and the difference in functional disability is minimized. Plasticity of brain can be utilized better through early intervention measures. The earlier you start better the outcome.

Brain circulation and vital centers.

Brain forms 2% of adult weigh but receives 20% of cardiac output and consumes 20% of oxygen supplied to the body. This shows its huge metabolic demand

- 10 seconds of blood supply disruption leads to loss of consciousness
- 4 minutes of interruption result in brain damage
- 10 minutes stoppage result in complete irreversible brain damage.

Brain is supplied through 2 separate set of arteries namely the internal carotid and vertebral arteries. All areas of the brain are important but some are more important to sustain life like brain stem, basal ganglia and grey matter. Generally, when body undergoes stress from shock it redistributes blood from non-vital areas (skin, muscles and GIT) to vital areas like brain, heart and kidneys. This is called diving reflex. Here some organs are compromised for the overall survival of the person. Brain gets better blood supply due to diving reflex. But inside the brain during shock, blood is redistributed to more vital areas of the brain (like brain stem, basal ganglia etc.) away from the less vital areas like white matter.

But if the shock is sudden like that occurring during cord prolapse or sudden placental abruption, there is insufficient time for this diving reflex to occur. In the absence of diving reflex the areas of brain receiving maximum blood supply suffers the most, i.e., brainstem and deep nuclei. After birth these babies present with more apneic episodes and less of seizures. Sudden blood supply disruption result in more brain stem damage and gradual and prolonged supply disruption result in more white matter damage.

Continuous supply of glucose and oxygen through undisturbed blood supply is the one crucial factor for the normal development of preterm brains. Compromised blood supply is otherwise called shock, and shock is the ultimate destroyer of tissues of all newborn brains. Newborns and preterm are highly vulnerable to infection and sepsis and it is the most common causes for shock.

Shock can be of different severity, intensity. It is broadly classified into uncompensated and compensated shock. Uncompensated shock (shock is present but compensatory mechanisms not working or inadequate) is usually severe and can be easily detected but is difficult to treat and ends in death very quickly if untreated. Other type of shock is called compensated shock whereby blood pressure is maintained at the expense of compensatory mechanisms of the body. These are the two broad classifications of shock but this is not enough if you analyze shock at a more microscopic level and its devastating destructions it can inflict. For more clarity shock is further divided into "subtle shock" where compensatory mechanisms have not been initiated or if initiated signs are less obvious, but some tissues in the body are having compromised circulation. For better identification and treatment of shock we need to reclassify shock in a better way. In older children and adults shock due to blood loss is well classified.

Types of shock:

Normal classification of shock is compensated shock and uncompensated shock. To get a clearer view on shock these two can be further subdivided into two subdivisions.

1. **Compensated shock**

    a. Subtle shock (subclinical shock, BP maintained)
    b. Compensated shock (BP maintained through compensation)

2. **Uncompensated shock**

    a. Uncompensated shock (BP not maintained)
    b. Terminal shock (Severe hypotension)

Table: 2.1: NYLE Classification of Shock.

Grades of shock	Common name	Signs and symptoms	Clinical implications
Grade-0	**Subtle shock** (Compensatory mechanisms not yet initiated or initiated but not clinically detectable)	Inappropriate color/dusky color for baby, CRT 2-3 sec, cold extremities, Irritable or lethargic child, mild metabolic acidosis or mild increase in lactate, apnea seen in pre-terms	Usually misses detection or detected when there is apnea, desaturations or seizures. Child can remain in this stage for prolonged period producing brain damage
Grade-1	**Compensatory shock** (Compensatory mechanisms initiated)	Tachycardia, tachypnoea, BP normal or increased, decreased urine output, metabolic acidosis & lactate increases, seizures, apnea, desaturations. CRT ≥3 sec, weak peripheral pulses.	Obvious clinical symptoms come up (this is the usual clinical detection stage)

Grade-2	**Uncompensated shock** (Compensatory mechanisms inadequate to maintain BP)	BP start to fall, compensatory mechanisms failed, seizures, desaturations	Panic stage, rapid deterioration and can rapidly go into cardiac arrest
Grade-3	**Terminal shock**	BP falls, bradycardia and cardiac arrest	Hopeless period, any time cardiac arrest

Table: 2.2: Stages of Shock and Clinicopathological Correlation

Grades of shock	Micro circulation changes	Damage is proportional to intensity & duration of shock	Neurological implications
Grade-0	Arterioles constricts & blood shunted from non-vital to vital organs, tissue level hypoglycemia & hypoxemia sets in and blood to vital organs is diverted from non-vital centers	Less intense but duration can be longer	Development of PVL, IVH (usually insults are not documented)
Grade-1	Compensatory mechanisms kick in, but microcirculation still suffers	Intensity of shock increases, duration variable	Higher grades of PVL and IVH
Grade-2	Compensatory mechanisms fail	More intense damage short damage	Major damage or +/− death
Grade-3	Circulatory failure	Intense damage	Major damage or +/− death

Facts about shock

Severity of brain damage is proportional to the severity of shock and duration of shock. So, severe shock of shorter duration can produce as much damage as subtle shock of long duration. It is common in NICU to find babies in subtle shock for long duration even for days without recognizing its significance only to produce higher grades of PVL and IVH, which is blamed on Prematurity. Prematurity never produces Periventricular Leukomalacia by itself, only additional insult occurring after birth is responsible for producing it. Finding the insult and preventing the damage is the real challenge and for that you need to have an open mind and needs to challenge some existing notions. Have you ever noticed, inside uterus no baby even with severe intrauterine insufficiency (IUGR) produces PVL at birth. It's all happening after birth.

Babies in subtle shock can go into apnea and desaturations. Babies should not remain in subtle shock or compensatory shock for long as some areas of the brain are definitely compromised during subtle or compensatory shock and that leads to damage. Recognizing signs of shock in its early stage (grade-0) is important in the prevention of brain damage. Proving this point is not easy through studies, but we can try treating shock with respect and see the change for your babies over time.

How is subtle shock producing brain damage?

Shock by definition is inadequate perfusion of tissues whereby supply of nutrients glucose and oxygen are compromised. A cell for its normal functioning needs continuous and steady nutrient supply and removal of its waste products. Main rate limiting nutrients and high turnover nutrients are glucose and oxygen. So, whenever there is slow perfusion the first to manifest are the deficiency of glucose and oxygen. Oxygen deficiency manifests as shift from aerobic metabolism to anerobic metabolism. Poor perfusion also results in glucose deficiency and cells experience tissue level hypoglycemia.

This cellular shift to anaerobic glycolysis is highly inefficient (16 times less efficient compared to aerobic metabolism; 2 ATP produced in anaerobic metabolism Vs 32 ATP produced through aerobic metabolism) (3). Due to this inefficiency, glucose requirement raises exponentially (Approximately 16 times more requirement, for producing an equivalent number of ATP). This glucose requirement cannot be met during this inadequate circulation. So, there will be **"Local Tissue Hypoglycemia (LTH)"**, which means blood glucose will be normal but at cellular level there will be hypoglycemia, since it is not easily measurable this is usually missed (all these years) and manifests later as tissue damage. On analysis you can see that the contribution towards this later damage is huge but remains hidden. The babies' blood glucose values may be normal or above normal but there is local tissue hypoglycemia.

During shock body is not able to supply glucose to tissues adequately resulting in tissue level starvation. A similar situation occurs in diabetic mellites, starvation in the midst of plenty. How to measure this tissue level hypoglycemia is the next big challenge. This tissue level hypoglycemia will be maximum where there is maximum decrease in perfusion and in tissues where utilization of glucose is maximum.

Most of the tissues (muscle, skin etc.) are resistant to tissue damage when perfusion is poor but can manifest if the circulatory compromise is severe. But brain, heart and kidneys are highly vulnerable to low perfusion. Brain because of its high glucose utilization rate manifests deficiency at the earliest. In the brain more vital areas are preserved (brain stem, basal ganglia, cortical grey matter etc.) at the expense of less critical areas like cortical white matter. Severe shock can affect any area. Subtle shock which can remain for long duration can produce havoc here without any dramatic signs and symptoms. The only signs and symptoms may be tonal changes, suppressed reflexes, lethargy, feed intolerance, irritability, apnea, poor color of baby or extremities, seizures etc. Subtle shock should never be left unattended and if on inotropes, doctor should not be in a hurry to stop inotropes unless doubly sure. There is a general tendency among doctors to stop inotropes quickly when NIBP is normal and if no gross signs of shock (tachycardia, desaturations etc.) are not there. Look for subtle signs of shock, including development of mild metabolic acidosis in VBG. The point is subtle shock can remain insidious for long periods (hours) before next ominous signs (apnea, seizure, desaturations) appear and initiate some actions. By this time the damage would have been done. Subtle shock produces damage to less vital areas like cortical white matter and presents later as PVL. This is my explanation for the poor outcome of a late referred sick baby from a peripheral hospital. Most of the time baby would have been in subtle shock unrecognized. They refer the baby when baby throws seizures, apnea, or desaturations. By the time baby comes to you most of the brain damage would have already been done. While treating shock we have to be aggressive in managing the underlying cause which in most cases would be an infection. Intensive care units worldwide are having the problem with MRSA, MDR & PDR gram negative organisms.

Subtle shock or subclinical shock (asymptomatic shock)

This stage of shock can be detected only by a well-trained eye. Its obvious manifestations are usually mild. So, you have to keep looking for subtle signs before any major manifestations like apnea, seizures, desaturations, sudden crashing of the baby happens. Most of the catastrophes seen in the NICU can be avoided if your staff is well trained to detect shock in its early stages. My hypothesis is that if you can prevent or treat babies in subtle shock properly then you can prevent brain damages like PVL, GM-IVH, development delay etc. At least you can decrease their intensity. We should approach shock in a baby like we approach compartment syndrome (CS) in thigh fracture. If we are diagnosing CS, it is already very late. Similarly, if the signs of shock have appeared, we are already very late.

Signs of subtle shock

- Bad appearance or dusky color for baby/mild peripheral cyanosis/baby not looking good.
- CRT borderline prolonged 2-3 sec, cold extremities.
- No signs of shock compensation like tachycardia, tachypnoea or hypertension [due to sympathetic and or Renin-Angiotensin – Aldosterone axis stimulation (RAA)]
- Usually mean BP will be maintained
- Child is either irritable or lethargic
- Mild metabolic acidosis developing with mildly increased blood lactate levels.
- Apnea, desaturations, lethargy, seizures, depressed neonatal reflexes.
- Feed intolerance like abdominal distension, altered RT aspirates, nausea and vomiting (↓ GIT perfusion).
- Decreased urine output (↓ renal perfusion).

When the baby is in its early stages of shock, cells are the first to experience the deficient supply of glucose and oxygen, they start to adjust by shifting to anaerobic metabolism and subsequently lactate starts to rise. But may be in its early stages tissues collective signals may not be strong enough to alert the higher centers like the sympathetic system to produce compensatory mechanisms. How does the higher center know that there is distress in the tissues? Most probably it is through the blood pH and other parameter like PCO_2, PO_2, HCO_3. As long as the blood pH is maintained in the normal range compensatory mechanisms don't get triggered. Once blood pH falls below a particular level compensatory mechanisms in the form of tachycardia, tachypnoea, rise in BP all happen and subsequently we are alerted. Lots of tissues need to get affected before it can alter the blood pH. When this much peripheral tissues are being affected then there will be compensatory mechanisms happening inside the brain also. There, blood is diverted away from the periventricular white matter to more vital areas like brain stem nuclei. It is not a hard and fast rule that only periventricular tissues are being affected, any areas can get affected. In short whenever peripheral circulation is compromised the CNS circulation is also compromised, if compromised circulation stays for long, unwanted manifestations can present later. This subtle shock can remain for hours or even days if there are no catastrophic symptoms to alert or if there are no doctors or staff who are smart enough to recognize it. We are usually alerted immediately when there is apnea, seizures, desaturations or if there is obvious shock. But if the protocol of that NICU for desaturations is to increase the FiO2 or for apnea if it is just stimulation or giving caffeine citrate without searching for its root cause then that baby will remain in subtle shock for prolong periods. For us a single apnea is enough for detailed investigations, upgradation of antibiotics (if required), and close scrutiny for shock. We invariable start inotropes at low doses (<10 mic/mt), which is also a good strategy to prevent further apneas.

Every neonatologist should self-analyze when did the baby had its first subtle symptoms and also the time elapse between the symptoms and any meaningful act towards it, is it hours or days! These are the precious moments during which unmeasurable damages are happening inside the brain. We have to be that precise in our actions then only we can match the quality of intrauterine environment. This kind of thing won't happen normally inside the uterus and no babies are born with PVL, GMH or IVH (but can happen when there is in-utero shock, sepsis or severe thrombocytopenia). Neonatologist will definitely act when there are signs of compensatory shock or if there is NIBP fall. Once there is BP fall then there is little time left before catastrophic events happens to the baby. Then we are at an edge of a cliff fighting for life. We should not corner ourselves into such situations.

When there is either manifested shock or subtle shock there is poor local tissue perfusion, correspondingly there is deficient supply of oxygen and glucose to the tissues. This creates local tissue hypoglycemia and damages the cells. But this is hidden behind the normoglycemia of the blood. The crux of this book is this tissue level hypoglycemia experienced by tissues during shock. I want to bring this idea into the open. This may be the explanation for the better neurologic outcome associated with HIE when accompanied by hyperglycemia. In severe HIE all kinds of insults can occur (hypoxemia, tissue level hypoglycemia, ischemia, seizure, sepsis etc.) and higher blood glucose improves outcome. Implying that cells would have undergone hypoglycemia during the HIE process even without blood hypoglycemia. By keeping higher blood glucose levels there is better outcome because of the better glucose supply to tissues during HIE. We can ensure better glucose supply by correcting the shock. The local tissue hypoglycemia produces its worst affects in tissues where metabolism is maximum that is in the brain. This **"undetected or subclinical shock"** produces local tissue hypoxemia and local tissue hypoglycemia which in turn produces neuronal damage. This may be the reason for the high prevalence of PVL, IVH, seizures in neonatal ICUs worldwide. **We are undermining shock and we don't have the specific tools to exactly measure it either.** We as clinicians should speak out our limitations and take a pledge not to undertreat any kind of shock. Till the time we invent exact techniques to measure subtle shock we should treat or overtreat shock to prevent thousands and thousands of cases of neurologically abnormal babies (PVL, GMH, IVH) worldwide. If this message is carried across, I am more than satisfied with this book. But everything needs molecular level proof. By giving better attention to shock we can drastically decrease the incidence of grade 3 or 4 IVH or advanced PVL. Our incidence of cystic PVL is almost nil unless cases are referred to us late.

One important point while treating shock is to take care of the primary cause producing shock aggressively which is invariably an infection. Now a days organisms are better armed and aggressive especially if acquired from our own NICU! Another important point while correcting shock is, compensatory mechanisms kick in and there is a chance for hypertension to occur and consequently there is a tendency to taper off inotropes prematurely, that is a self-made trap. Never aggressively taper inotropes during compensatory period of shock, even if you stop the inotropes at this stage BP will be maintained but that is for a short duration. Usually, compensatory mechanisms fail after some time if no corrective steps are taken and then you are into square one. During my 20 years' experience I have never seen any short term or long-term problems associated with hypertension occurring during the treatment of a shock. You can taper inotropes to a small extend when BP shoots more than 3rd centile values, never continuously taper and stop. Hyperglycemia is also a possibility at this stage but don't try to bring down glucose levels aggressively unless it is very high (>180-200 mg/dl) or is prolonged. Once shock and its primary cause has settled all these abnormalities will also settle on their own i.e., tachycardia, hyperglycemia, hypertension, tachypnoea, irritability, decreased urine output etc.

Always remember damage due to shock is proportional to the severity of shock and duration of shock. A preterm in subtle shock can remain for long duration until it produces dramatic signs or symptoms like apnea, seizures or till next consultant rounds the next day. This seizure and apnea are due to neuronal damage or neurologic dysfunction at microscopic level. Always treat shock aggressively with volume expanders and with inotropes and take care of the primary reason causing shock which is invariably an infection. A mild to medium dose of dopamine can do wonders to the baby, color and activity improves dramatically, and also need to upgrade your antibiotics if shock is not parting away.

> **Damage due to shock is proportion to severity of shock**
>
> **Damage due to shock is proportion to duration of shock**

All regular actions or events occurring in the world have a bell shaped gaussian distribution, people will be more focused on the middle 50%

of the values, problem comes when values are at the extremes which are usually neglected. In the case of shock, the subtle shock comes at the extremes of the bell-shaped gaussian distribution graph and its existence itself is questionable for many and manifest shock comes inside the middle 2SD. Everybody wants solid proof before initiating any action and are not at all bothered about the countless babies with neurological deficits. They want solid proof to link neurological abnormalities and subtle shock. Frankly speaking it is extremely difficult to prove this link through human studies as there are numerous confronting factors at play. Balancing two arms of a study group is a crude method of removing confronting factors. Each baby has thousands of its own variables and insults it had suffered while in NICU which are never measured or documented.

I am sure over the next decade it will definitely become a prime criterion of treatment to treat subtly shock by monitoring even mild accumulation of lactate. There is no obvious harm in overtreating shock at least in the initial phases. When to start, when to stop treatment of shock requires more scrutiny from clinicians. More micro analysis into the silent tissue level hypoglycemia during shock should be done. This book should encourage more thinking and studies in this direction.

Coming to the discussion on shock we have to redefine shock and its management to limit the neurologic damage. Shock should be viewed from a different angle, from cellular level, cells are the victims of poor perfusion. Shock should never be measured based solely on mean BP cut off values. We are not in a position to determine the level of tissue perfusion just by measuring mean BP alone. Also, we are not in a position to judge the tissue requirements of oxygen and glucose during shock. NIBP can be one of the parameters and not the only parameter. There should be more eagerness to start inotropes rather than to stop it. Knowing our limitations in measuring shock our cut off for mean BP is always 10-15 mm Hg higher than the set standard for the gestational age. To compensate for the low tissue delivery of glucose whenever there is shock or "subtle shock" or "poor perfusion" we have to keep the glucose value at a higher level, may be 100mg/dl or more. Values in the range of 50's and 60's need aggressive treatment. Otherwise, this becomes a double whammy.

What is the exact mechanism of neuronal damage?

Brain utilizes 20% of cardiac output that means it utilizes 20% of oxygen requirement of the body and similar percentage of glucose requirement of the body. Why the brain utilizes this high percentage of oxygen and glucose is due to its high metabolic rate. This very high metabolism is to maintain membrane polarity, cellular functions, neurotransmitter production, release and reabsorption. There are 100 times greater number of supporting cells executing various jobs. All require energy. A 10 seconds loss of blood supply produces loss of consciousness. This means that there are no energy reserves in the brain, continuous uninterrupted flow of blood (continuous supply of glucose & oxygen) is a must for the brain to function. In newborns whenever there is subtle shock the first area affected is the white matter areas of the brain where the capillaries carry less blood and correspondingly less oxygen and glucose delivered. Brain can revert to alternate fuels like ketones but their efficiency is very low, more over their supply is also restricted during shock. Maximum energy is required for the maintenance of cell membrane polarity through the action of Na-K ATPase. ATP supply disruption causes cell membrane instability, Na+ accumulates inside the cell and K+ outside. Sustained membrane depolarization occurs, increased intracellular Na causes activation of Na/Ca+ exchange and movement of Ca+ intracellularly in exchange for Na+. Additional crucial effects of this membrane depolarization are release of excitatory amino acids from synaptic nerve endings and reduced uptake secondary to failure of glutamate transport. The resulting extracellular accumulation of these excitatory neurotransmitters and consequent activation of glutamate receptors result in a variety of deleterious effects, including influx of Ca+. Calcium also may accumulate intracellularly because of failure of energy-dependent Ca+ transport mechanisms designated to maintain low cytosolic Ca+. The final common pathway to neuronal injury in hypoglycemia is similar to that in oxygen deprivation and relates especially to accumulation of cytosolic Ca+. More over in hypoglycemia, as in HIE, massive depletion of high energy phosphate compound does not appear to be an obligatory event producing cell death (9).

Considerable data indicate that the mechanism of cell death with HIE is mediated by the extracellular accumulation of excitatory amino acids, which are toxic in high concentrations. It also appears likely that excitatory amino acids play a major role in mediation of neuronal death with hypoglycemia. There are mechanisms for activation of apoptosis during hypoglycemia. Seizure can occur whenever there is shock due to the above-mentioned mechanisms. Sustained membrane depolarization and accumulation of excitatory amino acids are enough to trigger seizure during shock. In clinical practice we can see babies throwing apnea and seizures while in subtle shock.

Take-home message

- Treat shock aggressively and also sepsis.
- Detect and treat subtle or subclinical shock.
- Staying in compensatory shock is not good for long term neurodevelopment outcome.
- Severity of damage due to shock is directly proportional to the severity of shock and duration of shock.
- Classification of shock bring out subtle shock into limelight.
- Wherever there is shock there is associated silent tissue level hypoglycemia.
- Where ever there is a possibility of brain damage utilize plasticity of brain through early intervention measures.

Chapter-3

Tissue Level Hypoglycemia during Shock

Shock is a commonly encountered problem in the NICU and all are aware of its lethal consequences in its most severe form if not managed properly. But it is equally as lethal in its mildest form. This is the topic of discussion of this chapter. We have discussed different types of shock in the previous chapters, of which subtle shock is the least explored one.

A body distributes all its nutrients and oxygen required for the tissues through circulation. Normal glucose level is 60 to 120mg/dl and normal SPO2 level is 92-96% and cells gets affected when SPO2 falls below 90%. When the glucose level falls below 50%, Cells start producing distress signals manifested as lethargy, irritability, seizures, desaturations and the list goes on. So, the margin of safety of these main components of energy metabolisms are very narrow, that means the balance of demand and supply is very narrow. This is an indication that cellular requirements are very high even during resting state. When you exercise, (or when baby cries) the heart rate and respiration increase immediately to meet the cellular demands. So, we are normally living in the extremes and the reservoir function present in the body is minimal. We are in a dynamic equilibrium between demand and supply. Even the slightest disruption in the supply side can bring everything down.

Everything goes haywire when there is shock (decreased tissue perfusion). Shock in its advanced stages (compensated and uncompensated states) are well recognized by healthcare providers. If shock is left untreated baby goes into circulatory collapse or the baby throws seizures and ultimately dies. These are all known facts.

The scenario is different in case of subtle shock, it never leads a baby directly to death. Rather it manifests as apnea, desaturations, irritability, seizures etc. and doctors take remedial actions towards it. Before you take action, subtle shock can produce long lasting damages in the vital areas of the brain which are only manifest later.

Mechanism of cellular damage in subtle shock.

Imagine a neuron and its capillary blood supply. Under normal state neuron gets uninterrupted oxygen supply and glucose supply (main nutrients for the cellular energy production). During shock when the supply of oxygen is reduced cells shifts slowly into anaerobic metabolism and as a byproduct there is increase in blood lactate. Being highly inefficient in producing ATP its starts consuming more glucose molecules. Simultaneously during shock, the supply of glucose molecules into the interstitial fluid also gets reduced and neurons gets less and less glucose for its function. This deficiency of glucose during shock is called **"tissue level hypoglycemia"**. Simultaneous blood glucose levels will be normal or high, so this tissue hypoglycemia is masked by the blood normoglycemia. Proving such a hypoglycemia at a tissue level is not easy and so all these decades this was never identified. Subtle shock can remain undetected for hours so it can produce significant neuronal damage like extensive PVL, GM-IVH, microcephaly etc. More over during subtle shock the glucose requirement shoots up due to the inefficient anaerobic utilization. Anaerobic glycolysis is 16 times less efficient than aerobic metabolism (2 ATP produced during anaerobic metabolism Vs 32 ATP produced through aerobic glycolysis). Only external signal for such a shift to anaerobic metabolism happening inside the cell is the increasing blood lactate levels and development of metabolic acidosis. Usually this is missed because baby is relatively less sick and nobody bothers to do an ABG or a VBG, which are difficult and traumatic procedures. Clinically these babies can give subtle signs like poor appearance or dusky color of baby, borderline CRT, lethargy, feed intolerance, vomiting etc. These clinical signs are missed by an untrained eye. So, all of these neuronal damages can occur silently and never detected. But these babies on follow up can produce PVL of varying degrees on MRI but only to be blamed on the prematurity.

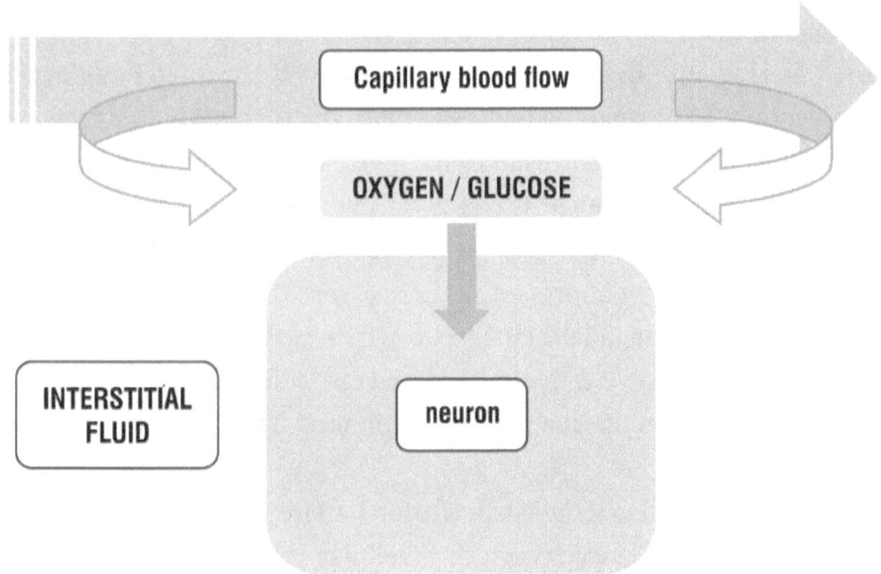

Figure: 3.1: Neuronal uptake of glucose & oxygen

Clearly speaking prematurity is not a cause for PVL, our inefficiency in treating premature babies properly resulted in PVL. That is the hard truth that we have to accept. Cells draws the glucose from the interstitial fluid and never directly from the capillaries. When there is an additional insult of blood hypoglycemia along with shock then the availability of glucose further deteriorates and the insult worsens. In the absence of shock, blood hypoglycemia is compensated to some extend by increasing blood flow. That may be the reason for the variation in symptoms of hypoglycemia at different blood glucose levels. A newborn may be perfectly normal without any symptoms with a blood sugar of 35 mg/dl and found out during routine GRBS screening. Some babies are symptomatic even at a blood sugar value of 50mg/dl. These are the babies likely to throw hypoglycemic seizures even at a glucose value of 50mg/dl.

Summary of different states

- Even during normal condition cellular requirements of glucose and oxygen are demanding, but when requirements are increased these can be met by increasing the local blood flow (arteriolar dilation).

- During pure hypoxemia, oxygen supply is disrupted but glucose supply is normal, in this case cells starts to shift to anaerobic metabolism. This results in increased glucose requirements and cells experience tissue level hypoglycemia. This increased requirement of glucose is met to some extend by increasing the local circulation, since there is no shock (for example by the arteriolar dilatation). But when hypoxia is severe, cells experience severe tissue level glucose deficiency in which case requirements of glucose cannot be met. This results in cellular damage.

- During shock (reduced perfusion) there is reduced supply of both glucose and oxygen and cellular requirements of oxygen and glucose cannot be fulfilled. Cells experience tissue level hypoglycemia and more over due to the associated hypoxemia glucose requirements increases many folds due to the shift to anaerobic metabolism. In this case there is high probability of cellular damage.

For the safety purpose in any sick baby keep blood sugar at a higher level (>80mg/dl). This is a protective mechanism because we cannot exactly measure the neuronal glucose uptake and the degree of associated subtle shock present. Cells undergoing hypoglycemic stress invariably produces stress signals to alert the body to improve the glucose supply. This stress response results in the hyperglycemia observed in some sick babies. Sometimes the center regulating blood sugar itself becomes the victim of tissue level hypoglycemia and produces inappropriate responses.

What happens when there is pure hypoxemia without any shock component? In this case glucose utilization by cells increases but they get adequate glucose through capillaries because there is no blood flow restriction. Blood lactate levels can increase without much cellular damage unless hypoxemia is severe. This is seen in congenital cyanotic heart disease babies where babies are comfortable with a SPO2 of 70-80% range (14). Same thing happens inside uterus where babies are comfortable with a PaO2 of 25 mm Hg which corresponds to a SPO2 of 45%. This point highlights the fact that shock is more devastating in cellular damage than hypoxemia alone, but both combined can have more damaging power. One thing is not clear why a normal person is struggling when SPO2 falls below 88-90% range and why a cyanotic congenital heart disease child is reasonably comfortable with a SPO2 of 70-80 % and why is in-utero baby so comfortable with a SPO2 of 45% (11, 12, 13).

As I have mentioned previously, cells cannot draw glucose directly from the capillary plasma and they have to depend on the interstitial fluid for glucose and other nutrients. When there is blood hypoglycemia, we treat with a glucose bolus which passes through the capillaries very quickly as a wave. Equilibration of capillary plasma glucose and interstitial fluid glucose takes on an average 8 to 10 minutes (10). This emphasizes the fact that bolus should invariably be followed by an appropriate glucose infusion. Babies who are under tissue level hypoglycemic stress produce neuronal metabolic derangements leading to firing by neurons to produce seizures.

Tissue level hypoglycemia during shock is a new concept and everybody reading this book should critically analyze this concept. Our next task is to find different surrogate markers to establish its existence and thereby monitoring babies based on that. During shock at cellular level the requirement of glucose skyrockets due to shift to anaerobic metabolism, so in any conditions where there is hypoxemia this phenomenon of tissue level hypoglycemia can occur. This can occur in cardiac and skeletal muscles during vigorous exercises. The cause of sudden cardiac arrythmia and death during vigorous exercise in some individuals may be due to this tissue level hypoglycemia on critical tissues and subsequent initiation of arrythmias. We need molecular level research to find out the truth.

Chapter-4

Which is More Damaging Shock or Hypoxia?

We all know that hypoxia and shock can both produce cellular damage. But we are not sure which one of these is deadlier. Over the years we are groomed to act swiftly when there is hypoxia (desaturation), and we are not that swift in action when there is a subtle shock. We are trained into believing that hypoxia is the main culprit and always worried whenever SPO2 is falling or is borderline. That is well and good because a falling SPO2 is an ominous sign. Detection of subtle or subclinical shock and its management has always been taken a backseat. This is because of the low awareness about the damages it can cause. There is a tendency among residents (reflective of consultants' attitude) to stop inotropes early in a sick child not knowing its consequences. During my practice we give inotropes for longer period until my child is completely out of sickness. I am aware that subtle shock is not easy to detect or measure, but can produce havoc if not given due respect. Neonatology over the years has improved dramatically. In well-established NICU worldwide neurologic outcomes are good. In ordinary set up the recognition of shock and its management are pathetic and so their neurologic outcome. The problem comes when these babies are referred to you (higher Centre) on day 3 or 4 of life when all these insults have already occurred and then you are in a mess, whatever great things you do nothing is going to improve their outcome. Most neonatologist are familiar with this kind of outcome. Even though there are tremendous advances in the field of neonatology the awareness and the devastating consequences of shock and early detection of subtle shock are still a distant dream.

In our NICU recognition and management of shock is aggressive. This has led to an excellent neurodevelopment outcome for our babies. Higher grades of PVL, IVH are very rarely seen. I attribute this to the better recognition and treatment of subclinical shock and its underlying causes.

How is hypoxia and shock fundamentally different? Both are a case of inefficient delivery of substrates to the tissues. Hypoxia is deficient oxygen supply to the tissues. While shock is insufficient perfusion of tissues leading to deficient supply of nutrient (glucose, amino acids etc.) and oxygen. During pure hypoxia there is adequate blood supply but with insufficient oxygen to tissues. This state is relatively better tolerated by most tissues (except CNS) unless SPO2 is very low and prolonged. Congenital cyanotic heart disease babies can tolerate pure hypoxemia better without much discomfort. They are comfortable with saturations in the 60's or 70's and they start to show discomfort when perfusion of tissues is also compromised (14). Fetus can also tolerate very low oxygen levels where saturations are in the 30's and 40's (11,12,13). To some extend this low oxygen content of blood is compensated by an increase in blood flow. The situation is very different when there is shock, during shock there is low perfusion into the tissues and so, not only oxygen but also glucose and other nutrient delivery to the tissues are affected. During shock there is no way to increase this nutrient and oxygen supply as autoregulation is nonfunctional in these tissues.

During shock there is arteriolar constriction and shunting of blood away from non-vital organ to vital organs. In the vital organs also, there is redistribution of blood from non-vital area to vital areas like brain stem and cerebral cortex. At any tissue level arterioles constricts and blood is diverted away from capillaries, capillary bed is where nutrient exchange is happening. Due to this blood diversion areas like periventricular white matter can suffer from ischemic damages. Measuring these subtle flow changes in these critical areas is nearly impossible in the near future.

Table: 4.1: Difference Between Pure Hypoxemia and Shock

Parameter	Physiology	Cells
Pure hypoxemia	Oxygen delivery to tissues is reduced but not totally stopped unless severe. Cells shift to anaerobic metabolism at some point. Glucose delivery preserved	Oxygen deficiency But Glucose supplies normal
Shock	Oxygen and glucose supply reduced; cells shift to anaerobic metabolism & tissues experience tissue level hypoglycemia. Anaerobic metabolism further increases glucose requirements.	There is both Oxygen and Glucose deficiency

When managing shock don't just go by capillary Refill Time (CRT) and mean BP alone as these can be deceptive. Mean BP may be the last value to fall and you may miss many cases of subtle shock. Look for the overall condition of the baby, look for the color, like a dusky color, any peripheral cyanosis, development of tachycardia, desaturations, apnea, feed intolerance, irritability turning into seizures etc. all these can be signs of subtle shock. Look for the development of lactic acidosis which are signs of anaerobic metabolism happening somewhere in the body. If baby's peripheries are not looking good means perfusion of tissues is not up to the mark and if that is prolonged other signs and symptoms can appear. It is better to assume skin perfusion as a reflection of CNS perfusion, if skin perfusion is compromised that means CNS perfusion is also compromised. Appearance of CNS symptoms will force you to act quickly. Incidentally skin and CNS develops from the same ectodermal tissue.

Shock by definition is inadequate perfusion of tissues there by nutrient supplies (oxygen, glucose etc.) are compromised. A cell to function properly nutrient supply should be adequate and so also removal of waste products (carbon dioxide). Main rate limiting nutrients (high turnover nutrients) are the glucose and oxygen. So, whenever there is inadequate perfusion the first to get affected are for the supply of oxygen and glucose. Oxygen deficiency manifests as peripheral cyanosis and shift from aerobic metabolism to anerobic glycolysis and manifests indirectly as appearance of lactic acidemia. This cellular shift to anaerobic glycolysis is highly inefficient in producing ATP {2 ATP (anaerobic) Vs 32 ATP (aerobic) metabolism so, 16 times less efficient compared to aerobic metabolism}. Due to this inefficiency glucose requirements sky rockets. (Approximately 16 times more requirement for the equivalent amount ATP production). This glucose requirement cannot be met by the already compromised circulation. So, there will be deficiency of glucose at the tissue level named **"local tissue hypoglycemia",** which means blood glucose will be normal but at cellular level there will be hypoglycemia, since this is not easy to measure it is always missed and manifests later as tissue damage. The baby's glucose value may be normal or high but there is local tissue hypoglycemia. Body is not able to supply glucose to tissues adequately (due to shock) resulting in tissue level starvation for glucose, starvation in the midst of plenty. How to measure this tissue level hypoglycemia is the next challenge new research into this is needed to find a surrogate marker for tissue level hypoglycemia. (Like lactate, which act as a surrogate marker of anerobic metabolism). So, when there is shock this local tissue hypoglycemia is marooned by the normoglycemia of the blood. **This may be the reason for the better neurologic outcome associated with HIE when accompanied by hyperglycemia (15).** This local tissue hypoglycemia produces its worst affects in tissues where metabolism is at the highest, that is in the brain.

During shock even without shift to anaerobic metabolism there is deficiency of glucose supply at tissue level, called tissue level hypoglycemia. shift into anaerobic metabolism worsens this glucose deficiency.

All kinds of shock namely **subtle shock (subclinical shock) or frank shock** produces local tissue hypoxemia and local tissue hypoglycemia which in turn produces neuronal damage. This may be the reason for the high prevalence of PVL, IVH, seizures in neonatal ICUs worldwide. We have to redefine shock and its management to limit the neurologic damage. Shock should be viewed from a different angle, from cellular level, cells are the victims of poor perfusion. Shock should never be measured solely based on the mean blood pressure (BP) cut off values. We are not in a position to determine the local tissue requirements just by measuring mean BP alone. How can a common BP values be the sole representative of perfusion when there is redistribution of blood at local level. BP cannot be one and sole parameters. BP is a general cutoff below which circulation can be compromised. Child can maintain BP by secreting counter regulatory hormones and activation of sympathetic systems which produces selective vasoconstriction maintaining BP. Knowing all these there should be more eagerness to start an inotrope rather than to stop it. Don't measure shock only through NIBP. Mean BP may be the last parameter to fall. Knowing our limitations in detecting shock, our NICU cut off for mean BP is kept 10-15 mm Hg higher than the set standard. To compensate for the low tissue delivery of glucose whenever there is shock or "subtle shock" or "poor perfusion" we have to keep the glucose value at a higher level. Be more aggressive when the blood glucose levels are in the borderline 50-60mg/dl range, accept higher glucose values during shock. This maybe the body's mechanism to compensate for poor tissue circulation.

When cells are suffering due to hypoglycemia is there a way for the cells to signal the body to increase glucose supply, or to increase perfusion? What is the cell's panic button? Cells have to convey to the body the difficulties it is encountering, for body to take remedial measures. If we can find this link and response then we can find signals for subtle shock. Is sympathetic stimulation the response of the body towards shock? (tachypnoea, tachycardia, hyperglycemia, peripheral vasoconstriction etc.). If so, we have to give importance to all signs of sympathetic stimulation very seriously.

One of the bodies mechanisms to counter this tissue level hypoglycemia is to produce hyperglycemia in the system as a whole. This may be the reason for a hyperglycemic response seen sometimes during sepsis, shock or seizures. Stress of local tissue hypoglycemia producing hyperglycemia in the child. Local tissue hypoglycemia gets buried in this blood hyperglycemic storm. When this counter mechanism fails to lift blood glucose level, hypoglycemia sets in which is the worst thing that can happen during a shock. So, shock associated with hypoglycemia is a deadly combination for neuronal damage. When there is tissue hypoxia manifested as raising lactate (acidosis), or when there is frank shock, you can be 100% sure that there is associated tissue hypoglycemia. That is why whenever baby remains in shock for some time child develops seizures which is actually **local tissue hypoglycemic seizure**. This tissue level hypoglycemia is marooned by blood normoglycemia. Tissue hypoxemia and tissue hypoglycemia go hand in hand during shock. Once cell's energy management goes haywire multiple mechanisms sets in for seizures like accumulation of excitatory amino acids externally, breakdown of Na-K ATPase etc. There should be an urgency to over treat shock rather than to undertreat it, as we don't know the limit of complete control of shock, there is no harm in over treating shock to save neurons.

I have wondered seeing some of the cystic PVL on MRI during follow up, how is it possible to produce such a large cystic lesion? A complete blockage of a medium sized arteriole can produce these punched out lesions, otherwise new explanations are needed. Severe acquired microcephaly seen in some babies are having homogenous damage throughout. Only a uniformly acting insult like hypoglycemia or shock can produce such a uniform damage. Tissue level hypoglycemia in shock is a good explanation for such a lesion.

In our NICU we always over treat shock rather than under treat it, because we don't know the exact boundary separating normal and shock. Our incidence of seizures, apnea is very low and moreover seizures are easily controlled if they ever occur and prescriptions of long-term seizure medications are a rarity. Incidence of higher grades of PVL, GM-IVH, apnea of prematurity is also very low. I attribute these good things to the better identification of subtle shock and its management. In my experience seizures are better controlled with inotropes rather than with anticonvulsants if you are treating the root cause. That mean it is very difficult to control seizure in sepsis (with subtle shock) with anticonvulsants alone and recurrence of seizures are very common if you don't take care of subtle shock. Recurrence of seizure is almost never seen if shock and sepsis are well taken care off. *(Anticonvulsant alone = seizure control difficult) (anticonvulsant + inotropes = seizure control easy).* Shock is mostly due to sepsis. The underlying primary cause also needs to be taken care of aggressively to get a success.

Coming to our chapter topic hypoxemia Vs shock, pure hypoxia as seen in congenital cyanotic heart disease is well tolerated, indicated by non-development of metabolic acidosis, non-triggering of sympathetic system, non-irritable child. This happens when there is no associated shock. Fetus can also tolerate very low oxygen. During pure hypoxia cell needs are met by varying the capillary blood flow, even though oxygen contend is less, supply can be increased by increasing the flow. Whenever shock component (deficient perfusion) enters the picture, supply of nutrients (oxygen and glucose) falls precipitously. Oxygen delivery to cells is never directly from hemoglobin to cells as discussed in the previous chapters. Capillary hemoglobin bound oxygen gets dissolved into the interstitial fluid from there oxygen gets into the cells. The solubility of oxygen in the interstitial fluid (water) is very less, so there is no reserve of oxygen in this interstitial fluid. The availability of oxygen is directly proportional to the capillary blood flow. Whenever flow is compromised supply of both glucose as well as oxygen are compromised. The conventional teaching stops by saying during shock there is deficient supply of oxygen and never discuss this deficient supply of glucose to the cells. This deficient supply of glucose is the damaging part, till now this component is unrecognized. Proving this concept through conventional Randomized control trials (RCT) is a waste of time as defining these are difficult. Only way is through animal studies in a laboratory.

In conclusion it is obvious that shock is more dangerous than pure hypoxemia. Be very vigilant when dealing with sepsis as detection of subclinical shock and its treatment is very important for the prevention of neuronal injury. Preservation of each neurons counts. The long-term neurodevelopment assessment (by measuring fine motor, gross motor, language etc.) seems very crude way of assessing brain function when you are thinking of preserving each neuron during shock. Preservation of all areas of the brain should be our priority. Aim should be **"intact survival"** rather than **"just survival"**.

> **SHOCK IS MORE DAMAGING THAN PURE HYPOXIA**
> **unless extreme**

Chapter-5

Is Subtle Shock the Hidden Monster in Preterm Brain Damage?

Clinical case scenario:

A preterm baby born vaginally at 29 weeks (1.36 kg), was admitted to NICU with moderate respiratory distress. Baby was put on CPAP for 72 hours and was administered surfactant, became off oxygen by day 6 and reached full feeds on day 10 of life. X-ray showed a picture of RDS, septic work up was positive and antibiotics was given for 7 days and **no inotropes were started**. There were two episodes of apnea requiring stimulation but no episodes of seizures or hypoglycemia during the stay. USG done on 7th day of life showed grade I-II GMH. Baby was transferred out from the NICU on 17th day of life and USG done at that time showed mild-moderate cystic PVL labelled as grade II-III PVL. This baby was discharged from hospital on 21ST day life. MRI on follow up showed wide spread cystic PVL. This is the usual picture seen in the many "not so high-end" NICU's in the developing countries. What happened in this case? was there any faulty treatment? or whether they have missed anything? My straight forward answer is that they would have missed the subtle shock. This is the usual picture seen in babies who had missed the subtle shock all together. This baby never had advanced stages of shock, which would have produced noticeable signs and symptoms which nobody can ignore. There are no other explanations for the moderate severe cystic PVL seen in MRI.

Whatever brain damage or developmental issues which prop up later are all dumped on the prematurity part or on ventilation if ever baby had undergone. It is like an accepted fact that all extreme preterm babies will have some form of neurological damage. This picture may not be true in developed countries or in top most NICUs in India. If that preterm was inside uterus and growing this would not have happened, so after birth we have done something terribly wrong to which we are not aware. Is it not our responsibility to find out the cause? Is this PVL preventable? My answer to this is yes to some extent, with little bit of more care towards subtle shock. Our baby must have experienced some degree of subtle shock for prolonged period which was missed by the caretaker. Baby also had apneas where subtle shock can be a reason. Retrospectively we cannot prove with hundred percent conviction, but tell-tale evidences are present.

Shock has well defined definitions and is always a common diagnosis in critical care units worldwide. Death certificates invariably show shock as one of its sub-diagnoses. We all have over simplified the concept of shock and helped it hide its ugly face. I doubt whether we are fully seeing the ugly destructive face of shock, my answer is a firm no. Major part of shock is hidden behind the tissue level. We are only seeing the above tissue level face of shock, that is, low BP, prolonged CRT, poor color, development of metabolic acidosis etc. Simple definition of shock is – circulatory system is unable to meet the tissue requirements of oxygen and nutrients. Main tissue requirements are for oxygen and glucose, which are simply an energy substrate and an igniting fuel (requirements for these go hand in hand). So, everything is all about energy requirements for running the cell, that is for running the Na-K ATPase pump, which consumes the maximum energy in a cell. Deficiency of which disrupts the cell membrane stability and integrity. Let us imagine shock as an iceberg with parts above the water (known to us) and with parts below the water (unknown to us).

Known facts about shock (Tip of the iceberg)

When a baby becomes septic, a multitude of chemicals are released by the organism and the body responds by producing "n" number of counter chemicals and mediators, some are useful, some are damaging to the body. Inflammatory mediators produce increased leakage from capillaries and fluid leaks out into the interstitial space producing generalized oedema and hypovolemia inside the vascular compartment. This hypovolemia is countered by secreting chemical which produces vasoconstriction. Kidneys start conserving fluid, clinically seen as decreased urine output. Stress hormones and chemicals released increase blood pressure. Body rationalizes blood flow by diverting blood away from non-vital areas to the more vital areas. So skin, GIT, muscles get less ration of blood manifested clinically as poor skin color, dusky skin color, prolonged CRT, hypotonia, tiredness. Decreased gut circulation may manifest as feed intolerance, altered aspirate, nausea, vomiting, abdominal distension etc. Vital organs get better blood supply but there also redistribution of blood happens. The blood is preferentially given to vital centers (brain stem, gray matter) at the expense of non-vital centers like white matter. Through these measures baby is trying to hang on to life by preserving function of heart, brain and kidneys. In that process it is compromising and damaging functions of other tissues which are not important for short term survival but important in long term. Babies' idea of maintaining BP at whatever expense is to save life rather than to protect each and every tissues. The counter measures improved perfusion pressure (BP), improved effective blood volume. This state is called compensated shock and is for short term survival as you have an array of tissues whose compromise led to the better perfusion of vital organs. So, it is obvious that this cannot go for long as these compromised organs start to demand their share or all these compensatory mechanisms crumble on to itself. During compensated shock white matter areas and lots of areas of brain are under stress. If this compensation remains for long severe brain damage ensures. So, whenever body tries to compensate and maintains blood pressure and circulation, we have to externally support the baby to relieve this compensation by giving normal saline push, starting inotropes and aggressively neutralizing infections by upgrading antibiotics. If you don't take care of infection part the cat and mouse game goes on and ultimately cat wins.

Converting compensatory shock into uncompensated shock occurs when BP starts to fall and all mechanisms for maintaining perfusion falls and then there is only one way that is the road to cardiac arrest. When blood pressure starts to fall blood supply to heart is compromised and heart starts failing and a vicious cycle set in and ultimately ends in cardiac arrest.

From this it is obvious that a baby should not be in compensatory shock for long, as there are compromised tissues and these tissues are crying for help. Not seeing their cry is like inviting trouble and later this cry becomes your scream.

Compensated shock: Signs and Symptoms

These are very well known to the readers and just recapping them for completions sake,

- Prolonged CRT, poor skin color, or dusky skin color
- Decreased and concentrated urine.
- GIT upsets like nausea, vomiting, poor appetite, abdominal distension, altered aspirates.
- CNS irritability, drowsiness, apnea, sometimes seizures
- Muscle weakness, tiredness, hypotonia.
- Development of metabolic acidosis, increasing lactate, desaturations
- Weak peripheral pulses and near normal central pulses, BP maintained.
- Development of tachycardia, tachypnoea, hypertension.

In short no baby should be in compensated shock for long, it is a ticking time bomb. How long is the question? I have in my experience seen many doctors not recognizing the subtle signs of compensated shock and happily continuing on compensated shock for long. This will either end in apnea, seizures or collapse of the baby or producing long term neurologic damage like PVL unknowingly. This is one of the mechanisms of developing neurological damage in neonates especially preterm. So, all the following signs should go before we can say there is no shock compensation.

- No tachycardia
- Normal CRT and NIBP
- Good color/appearance of baby, no cold extremities, child is active not drowsy, no hypotonia.
- No metabolic acidosis and normal range of blood lactate
- Non-irritable child
- Good urine output.

What is the role of inotropes?

Inotropes through its action on heart and peripheral blood vessels help to mitigate compensation and allow better perfusion of vital and non-vital organs. Sometimes when NIBP is normal even a low dose helps to improve microcirculations, babies' color/appearance improves, tachycardia settles, urine output improves, CRT normalization etc. can happen. My point is never going by BP measurement alone, if you go only based on NIBP values you will not start inotropes for majority of the babies initially, you will start inotropes only when condition worsens and by that time lots of damages would have happened. When you are handling a sick baby think in terms of tissue microcirculation whose deficiencies are manifested as subtle signs mentioned above. Do not be in a hurry to stop inotropes early, usually shock parallels sepsis and if sepsis is well controlled then your shock part will also be under control.

From experience I have seen that episodes of apnea in preterm babies are very less when baby is on low dose inotropes (dopamine 6 to 10 micg/kg/mt), consequently the use of caffeine citrate is also very less in our NICU. Our NICU neurodevelopment outcome for babies are excellent even without caffeine. Regarding apnea of prematurity my overall conclusion is that subtle shock or poor perfusion of vital brain centers has some role to play in its genesis. These vital premature centers are ultra-sensitive to perfusion changes. Diagnosis of apnea of prematurity (AOP) in pure sense should only be applied to extreme premature babies and not to babies more than 30 weeks. For babies more than 28 weeks before labelling as AOP make sure you are not missing subtle shock or any other standard causes.

So, in short identify compensated state of shock early and use inotropes more liberally. Try to be more vigilant to identify subtle shock and treat it. Always treat the primary cause which caused shock aggressively otherwise shock will return aggressively to haunt you. Better to over treat shock than to under treat it as we are not in a position to measure the ongoing damage of shock. There are no tools to measure damage caused by subclinical shock.

Always remember:

Compensated shock

> **= compromised shock**

>> **= compromised organs**

>>> **= organ damage**

>>>> **= cellular damage**

- Better to over treat shock than to under treat shock
- More liberal use of inotropes during shock
- Don't rush to stop inotropes
- Always be on the lookout for subtle signs of shock

Some unknown facts about Shock (Hidden Part of the Iceberg)

When we think or deal with shock, we only look at its gross parameters or gross manifestations, never into its inner cellular aspects. Let us go into more microscopic level of shock. Our body is made up of trillions and trillions of cells and our brain the most vital of all contains billions and billions of neurons and supporting cells. Shock effects all cells in the body, some are relatively resistant and some are highly vulnerable to changes to perfusion depending on its metabolic demands and cellular makeup. Neurons are highly vulnerable as they have very high metabolic rate. Constant supply of energy and fuel is a must for its smooth functioning. Any interruption in supply of these are instantly damaging and shock is the commonly encountered supply disruptor. Even during compensated shock there are plenty of areas of brain which are suffering. Don't be in the impression that during compensated shock all area of brain are well perfused. Aim of this compensation is to preserve life (by protecting vital brain centers and heart) rather than to preserve each and every tissue.

Microscopic view of Oxygen supply to tissues.

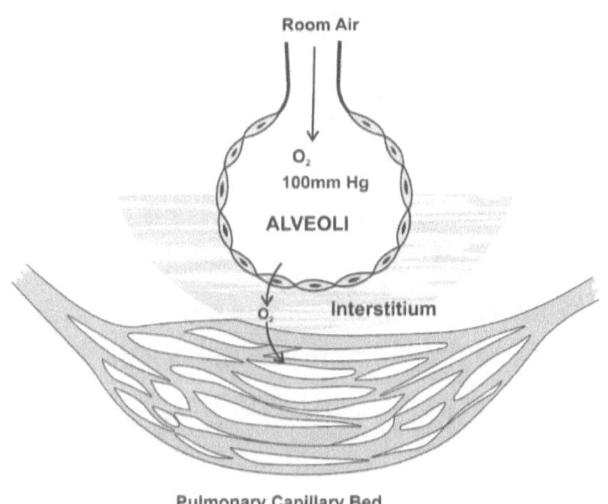

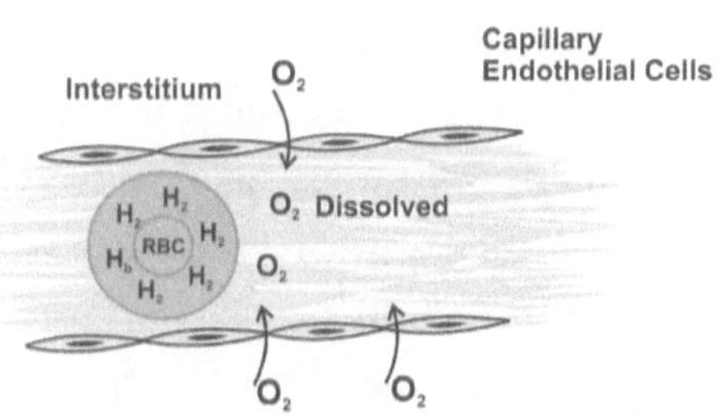

Figure: 5.1: Barriers and medium in oxygen transport.

Oxygen reaching alveolar space dissolves into the alveolar endothelial plasma, from there it goes into the surrounding interstitial fluid, from there into the pulmonary capillary endothelial plasma and then into the capillary blood plasma. Later majority gets bound to the RBC hemoglobin. A small fraction of oxygen travels dissolved in the capillary plasma. My point is oxygen never gets directly transported from alveolar space to hemoglobin in the blood, lots of fine barriers are present.

At the tissue end the reverse happens, oxygen from hemoglobin gets dissociated and through capillary plasma enters capillary endothelial cell plasma and from there it reaches interstitial fluid. Cells take up oxygen from the interstitial fluid. You can see there is no reserve capacity for oxygen in the interstitial fluid, oxygen supply and demand are in dynamic equilibrium. When supply is cut or reduced, cells feel the deficit instantaneously. Think about those vital neurons with high oxygen and glucose demand, any slight supply reduction is going to affect these neurons and its supporting cells. Neuronal supporting cell destruction (oligodendroglia, Schwann cells, microglia etc.) also affects neuronal health and its survival. Similarly, this continuous supply is required in the case of glucose also which is also in high demand in neurons, there is no reserve for glucose in the interstitial fluid. In short, any supply restrictions that occur during shock affects glucose and oxygen supply. Cells are starved instantaneously and shifts into anaerobic metabolism.

- No direct transfer of oxyhemoglobin to cells (only dissolved interstitial O2 enters the cell)
- No direct uptake of oxygen by hemoglobin from alveoli, always interstitial fluid is an intermediary for all O2 transport. (This may be a protective strategy against oxygen toxicity). The solubility of oxygen in water is very less so there is no oxygen reserve in interstitial fluid or plasma and thus, a continuous supply of oxygen should be there for the cells to survive.

- At the tissue end, dissolved oxygen in the interstitial fluid is the limiting factor for oxygen delivery to cells. When arterioles are constricted there is sudden drop in interstitial oxygen supply, since the solubility of oxygen is very low in plasma (water) the reserve oxygen available is extremely low and cells almost instantaneously experience hypoxemia.

- Analogous to oxygen supply, similar thing is happening in the case of glucose delivery. Cells also take up the dissolved glucose like dissolved oxygen, so when there is arteriolar constriction glucose supply also decreases. In short during compensated or uncompensated shock there is tissue level hypoxemia and tissue level hypoglycemia. In both these instances blood SPO2 and blood glucose levels are normal, concealing the tissue level deficiency. Of these only tissue level hypoxemia produces indirect signs of elevated blood lactate levels. There are no ways of detecting tissue level hypoglycemia with the present level of technology. We have to assume tissue level hypoglycemia whenever there is shock or whenever there is blood lactate elevation. So, shock means **"tissue hypoxemia and tissue hypoglycemia" which acts as a dyad, one is a substrate and the other is its fuel. It is logical to see when one is unavailable the other is useless.** When glucose is unavailable, the available oxygen is useless and vice versa until anaerobic metabolism kick starts. When anaerobic metabolism starts, glucose requirement shoots up due to the high inefficiency of anaerobic metabolism in producing ATP. Blood lactate level acts as a surrogate marker for anaerobic metabolism.

- What will cells do when there is tissue hypoglycemia. They try to utilize ketone as an alternate fuel. Alternate fuel supply of ketones is also not very high to fully replace glucose as the fuel. Moreover, they are also in short supply due to reduced blood supply.

Normal Oxygen & Glucose supply (without shock):

Arterioles supply blood to capillaries plentifully and so the arteriolar plasma oxygen and glucose contents are equal to capillary plasma oxygen and glucose, that is in equilibrium with interstitial fluid oxygen and glucose contents. Continuous uptake and supply of oxygen and glucose takes place. When the cell requirement increases there is arteriolar dilatation and supply increases. There are local tissue level regulators for these fine adjustments (autoregulation). This gets disrupted when there is shock.

Supply of Oxygen & Glucose during shock:

When there is shock, arterioles constricts and blood is diverted from less vital centers so, less RBC and plasma flow through the capillaries. The availability of hemoglobin bound oxygen and dissolved oxygen are less and correspondingly less dissolved oxygen reaches interstitial fluid. At the same time cells continuously uses whatever oxygen and glucose available in the interstitial fluid and soon end up in short supply. When oxygen supply is exhausted, cells shift to anaerobic metabolism and when glucose is exhausted cells looks for alternate source of energy. Since cells are drawing dissolved glucose and oxygen from interstitial fluid, there are no reserves for these and continuous capillary supply is a must for continuous tissue supply. This is a dynamic supply demand situation. During any kind of shock there is both deficiency of oxygen and glucose, which can be called **Tissue level hypoxemia and Tissue level hypoglycemia** (both these occurs in combination and this concept was not recognized previously). If you do blood glucose estimation at that time the blood glucose levels will be normal. The tissue level hypoglycemia is masked by the normoglycemia of blood. There is no way to measure tissue level hypoglycemia. When there is tissue level hypoxemia the cells shift into anaerobic metabolism and blood lactate levels rises and so lactate acts as a surrogate marker for the tissue level hypoxemia. In short, there is a way to measure tissue level hypoxemia but no way to measure tissue level hypoglycemia directly. We have to assume tissue level hypoglycemia whenever there is tissue level hypoxemia measured through increasing lactate levels.

During subtle shock or compensated shock, blood is diverted from non-vital organs to the vital organs. The blood is diverted from skin, GIT, muscles to heart, brain and kidneys. But the tissues from where blood is diverted don't suffer any damages, because these tissues have very low resting metabolic rates and are highly resistant to hypoxic damages. But the brain for which blood is diverted easily suffer ischemic damage during shock because of its very high metabolic demand. Normally 20% of cardiac output is consumed by brain. Any damage to neurons or its supporting tissues (oligodendrocytes, astrocytes, Schwann cells etc.) will have long lasting consequences. During compensated shock also the brain, heart circulations are not cent percent perfect and these tissues also suffer damages due to inadequate perfusion. Damage is time dependent. The longer these tissues experience compensated shock more will be the damage. So, damage due to shock is proportional to the duration of shock and intensity of shock.

Severity of damage due to shock is proportional to the

- **duration of shock**
- **intensity of shock**

Mild shock (subtle) for long duration is equivalent to intense shock of shorter duration. So, the following produces same damage:

- severe shock of shorter duration
- subtle shock of longer duration.

This relationship is important because staying in compensated shock is as harmful as uncompensated shock. Also remaining in subtle shock for hours is as harmful as compensated shock. Subtle shock recognition is poor in the untrained eyes, more so if awareness about its damage is not there. We tend to take quick action during severe shock as signs and symptoms are more intense and we may lose the patient if no action is taken. We have to be more vigilant and aggressive during compensated shock or subtle shock because the slow damage to cells (neurons) is always masked in the immediate period and manifests only later. This is very important in neonatal intensive care practice. Most damage to the preterm brain may be due to the overlooking of subtle shock for long periods or remaining in compensated shock. During compensated shock vulnerable areas of preterm brain – periventricular areas are deprived of oxygen and glucose and since there is no reserve for these substrates, the cells undergo tissue hypoxemia and tissue hypoglycemia. This causes ATP deficiency and can initiate several cellular adverse events like cell membrane disruption, enzymatic inactivation, accumulation of toxic products etc. all can lead to apoptosis. Preterm babies may remain in subtle shock for hours or even days {dusky skin color, peripheral cyanosis, slightly prolonged CRT (2-3 sec), mildly elevated lactate levels, ABG showing mild metabolic acidosis, poor activity, borderline SPO2, occasional apnea etc.}. This creates damage to white matter areas because of the compromised circulation, and later presents as varying degrees of PVL, overall reduces brain mass (microcephaly), ex-vacuo dilatation of ventricles and in long-term as diplegia, quadriplegia, cognitive deficits, seizures, etc. If you take a detailed history, you will not find any major insulting events like seizures, higher grades of germinal matrix hemorrhage, hypoglycemia etc. Natural question is why this PVL happening without major events? Usual tendency is to blame everything on the prematurity and escape. Missed subtle shock during preterm days were never blamed. That is why tissue level hypoglycemia has escaped detection for such a long time and now it is time to seriously bring out this culprit into the open.

For the better understanding of shock, shock can be better categorized into 4 grades namely subtle shock, compensated shock, uncompensated shock and terminal shock. Added 2 more grades to the existing classification were to get a better view on shock. In the existing classification of compensated and uncompensated shock, very subtle shock has no place. Terminal shock features are not clear. Terminal shock is just a march towards cardiac arrest and its progression is very fast and events occurring during terminal shock is very difficult to measure. The changes are exponential rise in acidosis (because of both metabolic & respiratory, pH drops very fast), rapid worsening of hyperkalemia and associated hypocalcemia.

Features of shock and its clinical applications.

Shock needs a reclassification because shock has various degrees of severity, it also helps to highlight subtle or subclinical shock better by keeping it separate.

Table: 5.1: NYLE Classification of shock

Grades of Shock	Common Name	Signs and symptoms	Clinical implications
Grade-0	Subtle shock	Bad color/dusky color for baby, CRT 2-3 or ≥3, cold extremities, Irritable child, mild metabolic acidosis or mildly increase in lactate, apnea for PT, feed intolerance etc.	Usually missed and child remains in this for prolonged period causing brain damage
Grade-1	Compensatory shock	Tachycardia, tachypnoea, BP increases, decreased urine output, metabolic acidosis increases & lactate increases, seizures, apnea, desaturations (R-A-A axis activation)	Obvious clinical symptoms come up (usual detection stage)
Grade-2	Uncompensated shock	BP start to fall, compensatory mechanisms start to fail, seizures, desaturations	Panic stage

Grade-3	Terminal shock	BP falls, bradycardia and cardiac arrest. Exponential rise of acidosis, hyperkalemia, and hypocalcemia.	Hope less period

Table: 5.2: Stages of shock and clinicopathological correlation

Grades of shock	Micro circulation changes	Damage is to duration & intensity	Neurological implications
Grade-0	Arterioles constricts & blood shunted from non-vital to vital organs, tissue level hypoglycemia & hypoxemia, in vital organs blood diverted from non-vital centers to vital centers	Less intense but duration can be long	Development of PVL, IVH (usually insults are not documented)
Grade-1	Compensatory mechanisms kick in, but microcirculation still suffers	Intensity of shock increases, duration variable	Higher grades of PVL and IVH
Grade-2	Compensatory mechanisms fail	More intense damage short damage	Major damage or +/− death
Grade-3	Circulatory failure	Intense damage	Major damage or +/− death

Most important aim of this classification is to bring out a clearer view on subtle shock which is usually hidden behind the bigger picture.

Grade-0 shock is the most important finding of this classification, the clinical findings about subtle shock is already known to everybody but my aim is to bring to light the damage it creates under the darkness. Grade – 0 shock is mostly undetected or not given much importance as long as it is not producing dramatic symptoms like apnea, seizures etc. or progressing to higher levels of shock. Even though the intensity of tissue hypoxemia and hypoglycemia is low, the duration it remains subtle shock is long to produce major damages on long term. During follow up it may present as varying degrees of PVL, IVH only to be blamed on prematurity. Retrospectively no major insulting events may be recorded.

For controlling shock, importance should be given for the primary cause. Invariably the reason for shock will be a sepsis and if sepsis is not treated properly shock will never get under control. A shock is fully controlled when you don't have any of its compensatory mechanisms seen (no tachycardia, no metabolic acidosis or tachypnoea) and child is look very active, no apnea or desaturations, normal CRT etc. At this stage there will not be any arteriolar constriction and no shunting of blood from one region to other and no cellular shift to anaerobic metabolism. Only a near total hypoxemia can push a cell to death, cells can survive with a PaO2 as low 1 mm Hg (16). Simultaneously occurring tissue level hypoglycemia during shock is the real damage maker. In conclusion shock seems to be the silent damager of brain especially in preterm and newborn brains. Subtle shock recognition and treatment need more attention. We have to be extra cautious when dealing with sepsis and shock. Yes, subtle Shock is the Hidden Monster in Preterm Brain Damage.

Chapter-6

Does Tissue Level Hypoglycemia Always Accompany Shock?

Shock is a common occurrence in ICU's all over the world. Shock is usually associated with deficient supply of oxygen and nutrients, but the nutrient factor is never highlighted or given any importance. Even if discussed it is only in association with blood level hypoglycemia. Never had the discussion of tissue level hypoglycemia in the setting of blood normoglycemia. If you have understood the full mechanisms occurring during shock from the previous chapters, it is obvious that hypoglycemia invariably accompanies shock. Due to arteriolar constriction and diversion of blood there is deficiency of both oxygen and glucose as there are no reserve of these (oxygen & glucose) both inside and outside the cell. Oxygen solubility in plasma is very less, so also is the available glucose in the plasma or interstitial fluid. Both oxygen and glucose are in dynamic equilibrium with the cellular consumption. Unmeasurable nature of tissue hypoglycemia makes it undetectable or nonexistent. You can assume that if there is development of metabolic acidosis due to poor perfusion then you can be sure that there is tissue level hypoglycemia. As soon as there is shift to anaerobic glycolysis the efficiency of ATP production reduces by 16 times and correspondingly glucose requirement shoots up 16 times but supply of that much glucose is not possible in the setting of shock (2, 17). We can conclude that there is definite tissue level hypoglycemia associated with shock unless proven otherwise.

Roughly 10^9 molecules of ATP (1 billion molecules) are in solution inside a typical cell at any instant and this ATP is cycled in every 1-2 minutes (18). So continuous supply is a must in highly active cells and is very much true in case of neurons. That is why damage is instantaneous once there is short supply of blood. Oxygen usage is linked to glucose consumption and as soon as oxygen deficiency causes shift to anaerobic metabolism, the consumption of glucose shoots up due its inefficiency. Meeting the cellular requirements is nearly impossible. Shifting to ketone metabolism is also not possible because in shock its availability is also reduced.

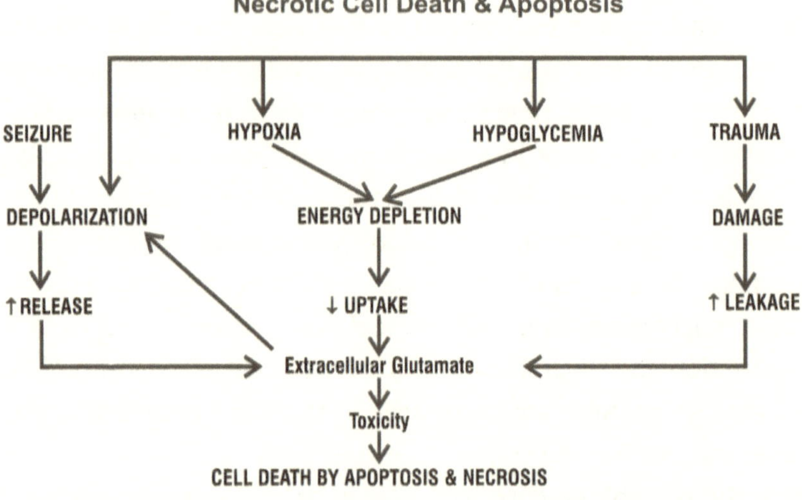

Figure: 6.1: Necrotic Cell Death & Apoptosis

A complete stoppage of blood supply to brain for 10 seconds makes a person unconscious and 3-4 minutes stoppage can result in death. This shows the dynamic nature of the energy and substrate requirement of brain. I wonder why hypoglycemia was never considered during shock. HIE studies had given us a hint in the form of better neurologic outcome seen in cases with hyperglycemia. We didn't take this leed to its finer analysis. So just higher glucose levels were enough to produce better outcome, this shows the dependency of neurologic outcome on the blood sugar values. If the blood sugar values are higher cells would get a bigger proportion of glucose. It can be assumed that hypoglycemia associated with shock can be a deadly combination.

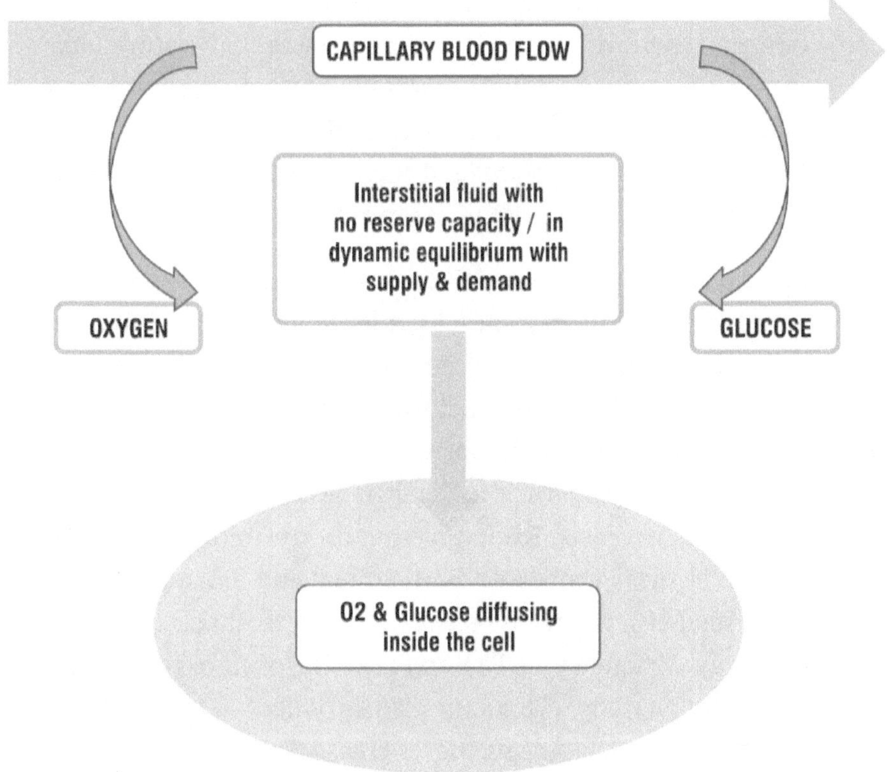

Figure: 6.2: Oxygen and Glucose transport at cellular level.

Features seen at the tissue end of capillaries.

- Constant supply of oxygen and glucose into the interstitial fluid from the capillaries.
- Constant uptake of oxygen & glucose by the cells
- Supply and demand are in dynamic equilibrium
- Any supply disruptions at capillary end (during shock) instantaneously pushes interstitial fluid into deficit

- As long as there is no shock demand is met by the capillaries.
- Oxygen supply disruption leads to shift to anaerobic metabolism which increases glucose demand 16 times for the equivalent ATP production.
- This means that under no circumstances one should allow the shift to anaerobic metabolism. That may be the reason for giving oxygen whenever there is shock even though saturations are in the high upper limits. Anaerobic shift drains out whatever glucose is available in the interstitial fluid.
- During shock tissue or cellular level hypoglycemia is a common occurrence similar to tissue hypoxemia.

Hypoxemia and hypoglycemia lead to energy depletion and depolarization of cell membranes. This leads to decreased uptake and increased release of excitatory neurotransmitter glutamate, which in turn causes toxicity to the neurons. Toxicity leads to apoptosis or necrosis of cells. When the insult is a slow there is more chance for apoptosis to occur and if the insult is acute and severe there is a more chance for necrosis. Excitatory neurotransmitter glutamate has a central role in these processes. Both animal and human studies have confirmed this (19). So, in hypoglycemia and in shock there is both cellular energy deficiency (ATP) and toxicity from excitatory amino acid glutamate. Glutamate toxicity also produces seizure which can aggravate the insult. Seizures further increases energy requirements.

In conclusion treat shock at any cost and consider associated tissue level hypoglycemia with shock. Maintain a higher blood glucose preferably >100mg/dl when associated with shock. (Needs further studies to find out the best glucose values during shock).

By giving oxygen during shock though nasal canula or mask, it increases dissolved oxygen content in the pulmonary blood vessels and that dissolved oxygen directly reaches the capillary bed of tissues and dissolves into interstitial fluid of tissues. Only dissolved oxygen in the interstitial fluid is available for cells. So, this extra oxygen (in the form of dissolved oxygen) directly reaches cell. While the RBC hemoglobin bound oxygen will be replenishing the capillary plasma oxygen, which subsequently diffuses into the interstitial fluid. There is no direct transfer of Hb-bound O2 into the interstitial fluid. That is why any sick baby suddenly improves if you give oxygen even when saturations are in the normal range. Dissolved oxygen status improves (by giving extra oxygen) and it directly supplies oxygen to all the cells of the body.

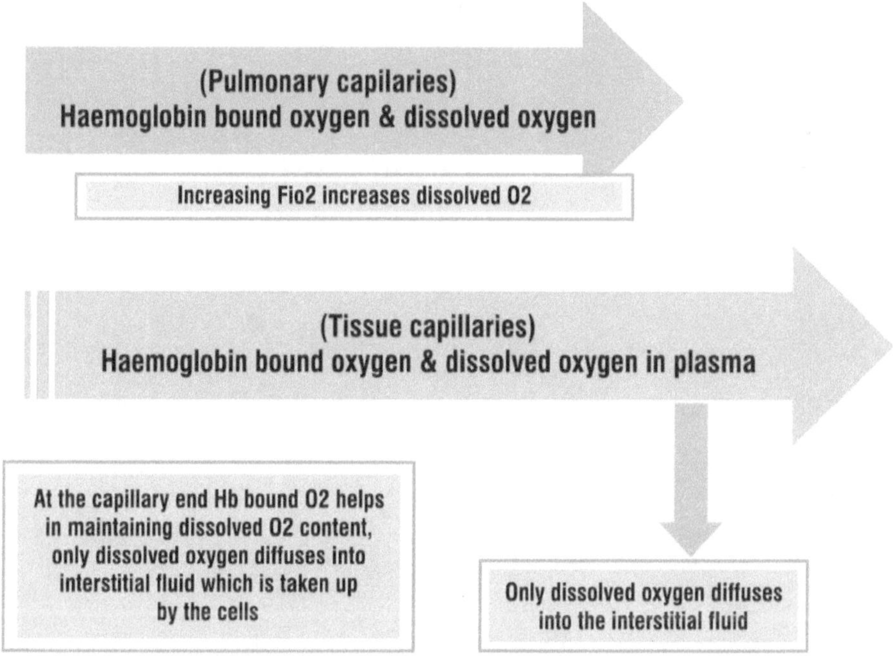

Figure: 6.3: Oxygen diffusion at capillary end

Chapter-7

Apnea as a Manifestation of Early Shock in Preterm

Can apnea be a manifestation of early shock in preterm babies? Can early inotrope administration prevent apnea?

In this chapter we will discuss the relationship of apnea and early shock or subtle shock. Definitely shock can manifest as apnea in preterm babies. By using inotropes early and with appropriate management of subclinical shock apneic episodes can be controlled to some extent.

Case scenario

A 30 weeks old preterm baby admitted to NICU showed 2 episodes of apnea on day 3 of life. Baby was on caffeine citrate since day 1 of life and later the frequency of apneic episodes increased and had to ventilate the baby on day 4 of life. Septic work up turned positive on day 4 of life even though initial workup was negative. By this time child had prolonged CRT and other clinical signs of shock. Inotropes and higher antibiotics were started and baby improved and extubated on day 8 of life.

Discussion:

This is a common scenario seen in NICU and is a clear case of sepsis and shock producing apnea as an early sign. Mostly we take this as apnea of prematurity, but Apnea of prematurity (AOP) should be a diagnosed only after excluding other causes. In this case apnea may be the first manifestation of subtle sepsis and shock sequence and no other signs may have appeared clinically or clinical signs was overlooked.

Sometimes a closer look may reveal subtle perfusion deficiencies and septic work up may or may not be positive.

Early initiation of low dose dopamine (5-10mcg/kg/min) and normal saline bolus and upgrading of antibiotics would have prevented ventilatory requirements. Apnea definitely can be a manifestation of early shock. The brain stem vital centers would have undergone subtle perfusion abnormalities and the resulting energy failure (tissue level hypoglycemia) and accumulation of excitatory amino acids all can manifests as apnea and sometimes even as apneic seizures. Just starting inotropes can prevent further apnea episodes but always take care of the primary cause which in most cases will be an infection or an electrolyte abnormality. If no action is taken towards sepsis or electrolyte abnormalities the inotrope requirements progressively increases and apnea recurs. Apnea occurring anytime should prompt a thorough workup to rule out sepsis, electrolyte abnormalities and a Neuro-sonogram (+/− LP).

Apnea of prematurity (AOP) is seen in premature babies below 34weeks. But strictly speaking it should only be applied in babies less than 30weeks gestation (personal opinion). Older babies can also have apnea but usually due to some definite causes. Babies below 30 weeks can have apnea without other causes and can be rightly called apnea of prematurity, but investigation to rule out other causes should be done. Do other babies with apnea who are >30 weeks have the right to be called apnea of prematurity. My personal opinion is no, because they have some other additional problems which tripped them into apnea. We have to find that cause, mostly it is a shock, sepsis, IVH, PVL, GMH, metabolic acidosis, electrolyte abnormalities, or a NEC. In sepsis and shock, apnea can be an early manifestation. In our NICU the use of caffeine citrate for apnea of prematurity is very less for babies more than 30 weeks. I see apnea as a manifestation of poor brain stem perfusion (shock) before other signs and symptoms manifests. We use more of low dose inotropes for preterm babies rather than caffeine citrate for prevention of apnea.

Caffeine citrate actually increases left ventricular output in preterm infants by a combination of positive inotropic and chronotropic effects (20). Caffeine, by increasing left ventricular output in a way acts like an inotrope. Better long-term neurodevelopmental effects of caffeine may be due to this better perfusion of tissues. Our incidence of apnea in NICU is very less and so are other neurological deficits. This is a tectonic shift in thinking and will take years before it will be appreciated. I encourage doctors to apply this principle in patients and see the positive results. For seeing success, you have to coverup the sepsis part properly. Proving through RCT is indeed needed but due to so many confronting factors this may end up equivocal. Most difficult part in this is the proving of sepsis which in most cases may end up as septic screen negative.

How is apnea produced?

You have the respiratory center in the brain stem controlling respiration. It has afferent impulses (sensory) coming from different areas of brain and from respiratory and cardiovascular system. Based on inputs like blood pH, PCO_2, PO_2, HCO_3 etc. respiratory center controls the rate and depth of respiration. There is a time lag between input and output signals and this is more pronounced in preterm babies. In preterm babies all centers involved are immature and shows waxing and waning effect and any additional insult can prolong the waxing and waning effect, manifesting as apnea. Due to immaturity any slight insult is enough to derange the functions. Changes like blood pH, perfusion disturbances, hypoglycemia, seizures, electrolyte abnormalities, opening up of PDA and its circulatory changes, sepsis, pneumonia all can lead to apnea. Since infection in preterm babies is a common problem, sepsis and shock are a common precipitating factor for apnea. Due to multitude of factors, subclinical shock is a common accompaniment during infections. Prompt and appropriate action at this stage can save you from more troubles like intubation and ventilation. When apnea occurs first rule out other causes and then only label it as AOP, otherwise you are into trouble.

In extreme premature babies also, before labelling apnea of prematurity rule out other associated causes. In these infants, perfusion changes can occur even without infections. In preterm babies because of the immaturity of the respiratory center (myelination not complete, neurotransmitter production and recycling not mature, specific neurotransmitter dominance may not have attained, pathways for input and output signals may not be fully myelinated etc.) might make it highly vulnerable to external influences like pH, electrolyte oxygenation variations, inflammatory mediators etc. (21).

Respiratory center processing can be affected in different ways

- Altered perfusion related

    - Sepsis, shock, hypoxemia, tissue level hypoglycemia and energy failure
    - Altered blood pH related respiratory cell depression
    - Accumulation of excitatory amino acid and abnormal firing

- Abnormal afferent impulse from brain (seizure) or periphery (chemical sensory impulse – pH, PCO2, HCO3, PO2, other impulse from GERD, NEC, pneumonia).
- Other systemic insults on respiratory centers

    - Electrolyte abnormalities
    - Hypoglycemia
    - PDA and its hemodynamic effects
    - IVH, GMH, PVL, meningitis

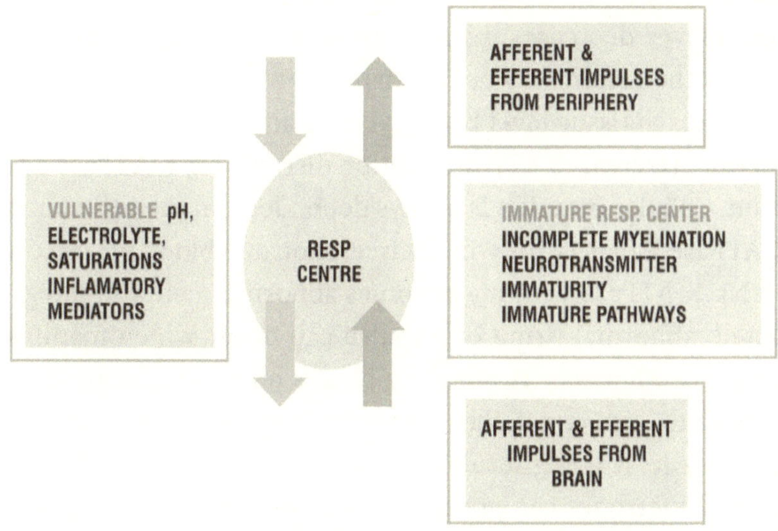

Figure: 7.1: Respiratory center and its vulnerabilities.

Apnea can be a manifestation of "n" number of diseases and the discussion will be restricted to that of shock. Most sick babies in NICU will have sepsis as part of their diagnosis. AOP is a diagnosis of exclusion unless the baby is extremely premature like that of 30 weeks or less. More mature babies if all the vital parameters are fine and if there are no signs of sepsis, shock, PDA, NEC, electrolyte abnormalities, IVH, GMH, or PVL should not have apnea. For these babies any additional insult can push them into apnea. But as the baby becomes more mature, they attain more resistance towards these precipitating factors. After 34 weeks these factors are less likely to precipitate apnea unless the insulting factors are severe. After 30 weeks of maturity do not consider AOP as the first diagnosis, exclude all other factors first. While excluding look for subtle shock carefully (poor color of baby, dusky skin, slightly prolonged CRT, mild metabolic acidosis, decreased urine output, increasing blood lactate levels etc.). You have to train your eyes properly to find subtle shock.

Preterm baby's respiratory center is highly sensitive to changes to the blood pH, PCO2, PO2, and electrolytes. So, whenever there is poor perfusion, blood lactate accumulates and pH starts to drop, oxygen deliver decreases, so also tissue delivery of glucose. Can all these alter the respiratory center firing? Decreased tissue delivery of glucose leads to tissue level hypoglycemia and decreased cellular ATP production. Decreased ATP production disrupts Na-K ATPase enzyme function. Cellular function is always dependent on the cell membrane Na-K ATPase integrity for which circulation and blood pH are crucial. When Na-K ATPase working becomes abnormal, cell wall integrity is disrupted, abnormal firing of impulse can occur which manifests as seizures. So, whenever respiratory center microcirculation becomes inappropriate, energy failure ensures, which causes apnea and abnormal cellular firing resulting in seizures. Controlling shock early and adding inotropes can prevent further deterioration of apnea. Use inotropes for sufficient period of time before sepsis is well under control. These same mechanisms help in better perfusion of other parts of preterm brain and thus can avoid getting PVL, IVH, GMH etc. Our unit has very low incidence of serious PVL, IVH, GMH and this may be due to the "over use" of inotropes. Microcirculation abnormality is the real cause of brain damage. There is no direct method to measure microcirculation, now people are using lactate as a marker for that, I use the clinical method of color and appearance of baby, CRT and lactate levels for the monitoring of subtle shock. One practically useful rule is **"if skin circulation is bad, CNS circulation is also bad and if skin circulation is good then CNS circulation is also good"** – after all both develop from the same ectodermal tissue. If babies' skin appearance is not good that means babies skin circulation is compromised for CNS circulation and this compensation is not good in the long run. If baby is making some circulatory adjustments that means the overall circulation is not good. This microcirculation failure can cause apnea later. Help the baby at this stage to tide over the situation.

In short, apnea can be a manifestation of lots of conditions and one of them is early shock. Try out these in your practice to see its correctness.

Chapter-8

Can Seizure be a Manifestation of Shock?

Shock is a common manifestation in neonatal and pediatric practice. There are several causes and mechanisms for shock. Any sick neonate can throw seizure at any time. My experience over the years had taught me that shock is a prominent mechanism causing seizures in a sick-septic baby. This strategy of treating subtle shock along with anticonvulsants to control seizures have given me great dividends. In this discussion I am not considering epileptic seizures, febrile seizures or other known seizure syndromes. Only discussing seizures occurring in a sick septic baby in a neonatal ICU.

Case scenario

A 4-day old newborn was brought to the NICU from postnatal ward with respiratory distress, poor perfusion, desaturations and tonic-clonic seizures. Baby was 3.5 kg at birth and was feeding well until yesterday in the wards but had mild lethargy. But on morning rounds was found to have seizures and respiratory distress. Septic work up done was positive and X-ray showed pneumonic patches. Child had prolonged CRT and low BP. Baby was treated in NICU with IV antibiotics, anticonvulsants, Normal saline push, inotropes and oxygen. Child improved and went home on 10th day of life; CSF analysis and neuro-sonogram was normal.

Discussion

This is a usual presentation seen in the postnatal wards and all are familiar with this type of presentation and its management. But this case can be mismanaged in "n" number of ways. Have you ever thought about the mechanisms of seizure in such cases?

Probable mechanisms of seizure.

1. Seizure can occur due to the release of massive amounts inflammatory mediators from infection.
2. Hypoxia of neurons leading to ATP deficiency and membrane Na-K ATPase disruption.
3. Due to blood hypoglycemia and subsequent cellular energy failure.
4. Shock related mechanisms.

    a. Hypoxemia to cells
    b. Tissue level hypoglycemia accompanying shock (mechanisms discussed in previous chapters)
    c. Energy failure leading to persistent depolarization of neurons triggering seizures.
    d. Electrolyte abnormalities (hypocalcemia, hypo and hyper natremia) can trigger seizures.
    e. Energy failure leading to the accumulation of excitatory amino acid externally leading to seizures.
    f. Apoptosis and necrosis of neurons from multiple mechanisms

Severe sepsis can cause massive release of inflammatory mediators which can cause seizures. Since LP and USG head were normal, causes related to these were not considered. On analyzing closely, we can see that shock has a major role to play in seizures. During shock there is diversion of blood from non – vital centers to vital centers. Non-vital centers like periventricular white mater suffers, and in severe shock other centers also suffers. Subtle shock of long duration makes the same damage like severe shock of shorter duration. As explained in other chapters on shock there is energy deficiency to the cells from hypoxemia and tissue level hypoglycemia. Due to the energy deficiency, cell membranes are persistently depolarized, there is decreased uptake of excitatory amino acids, which can trigger seizure. Apoptosis and necrosis caused by multiple mechanisms can also led to seizures.

On microanalysis of sepsis and shock we can see that there is deficient supply of glucose and oxygen to the cells. In neonatal period shock is a leading cause of seizures. Early recognition and treatment of shock can prevent seizure. There is a high chance for missing early shock in postnatal wards and even in NICU's.

Chapter-9

Analysis of Blood Hypoglycemia and Shock (Tissue level Hypoglycemia)

Blood hypoglycemia is a common occurrence in neonatology and symptomatic hypoglycemia can produce long term neurologic damages in babies. The value at which a baby develops symptoms of hypoglycemia is highly variable, let us take a typical example of a newborn case of hypoglycemia occurring in a postnatal ward. For a 3kg baby the following values can be assumed.

- Blood sugar >60-100 mg % normal
- Blood sugar 60-50 mg % borderline normal
- Blood sugar 50-40 mg % borderline hypoglycemia
- Blood sugar <40 mg % definite hypoglycemia

The level at which baby produces symptoms vary depending on how closely you are watching, some symptoms are obvious like seizures, lethargy, severe jitteriness. But some symptoms and signs are subtle like mild lethargy versus sleepiness, mild jitteriness, mild tachycardia which can occur normally also, So, the line separating asymptomatic hypoglycemia and symptomatic hypoglycemia is very much blurred. If you analyze the above values, you can see that a baby can be perfectly normal at blood sugar values above 60 mg % and the same baby start showing symptoms when blood sugar value dips below 50 mg % and any time baby can throw seizure. So, the baby is working on a thin margin of safety of only 20 mg, doesn't it seem surprising? Every baby is living on the edge and the margin of safety for several factors are very thin. There is a high variability among babies on the subject of which symptoms to produce and when. In this ultra-thin line of separation of normoglycemia and hypoglycemia, imagine what shock can produce in this situation. Shock even in its subtle form can reduce the glucose and oxygen supply significantly to an area and immediately produces tissue level hypoglycemia. There is instantaneous deficiency of glucose and cell functions are disrupted and cellular firing and seizures can occur. The intensity of shock may vary in different regions of brain producing different symptoms. One thing is clear shock and blood hypoglycemia combination is a deadly combination. Once you understand the mechanism of shock well, shock seems synonymous with tissue level hypoglycemia. blood hypoglycemia and tissue level hypoglycemia produce same cellular damage.

Once you understand the mechanisms operating behind shock you have to be ultra vigilant against shock, this is not to spread panic among doctors but to bring awareness on the devastating damage it can produce on babies. Until and unless we are perfect with the knowledge of neuronal damage, we have to be vigilant against tissue hypoglycemia (shock) and blood hypoglycemia.

Chapter-10

Blood Hypoglycemia & Tissue Level Hypoglycemia

It is a common knowledge that there are variations in the levels at which newborns produce symptoms of hypoglycemia, moreover the type of symptoms varies greatly. Individual babies have their own cut offs for producing symptoms during hypoglycemia. Some babies are perfectly asymptomatic even with a blood glucose value of 30-35 mg/dl. Some babies through away seizures even at a blood glucose value of 50-55 mg/dl. Several explanations can be seen in text books. Cells experience hypoglycemia when there is absolute fall in blood glucose level or when there is perfusion deficiency (shock) with normal blood glucose levels. Sometimes both these can occur simultaneously i.e., shock associated with low blood glucose.

A cell can experience nutrient deficiency (glucose or oxygen) either due to

- Deficient circulation (perfusion)
- Low absolute value of nutrient in the blood or in the interstitial fluid surrounding a cell.

Normal average cerebral blood flow in adult humans is approximately 50 ml/100g/minute. In white matter it is 20 ml/100g/min and in grey matter it is 80 ml/100g/min (1).

Placental blood flow is 600 to 700 ml/min, for a 3 kg term fetus it is about 200-230 ml/kg/min (11,12,13). When compared, in adult it is 5 liters/min, converting to per kg, for an average 70kg person it comes to about 72ml/kg/min. Comparing placental output with cardiac output the ratio comes to about 3:1 (placenta: adult). That means placental blood is circulating 3 times faster than in adult. In placenta blood oxygen partial pressure is 3 times less than (Umbilical vein PaO2 of 30-34 mmHg) in adult aortic blood oxygen tension (i.e., 100 mm Hg). In circulation when nutrient value is low, it is compensated by an increase in the circulation. This autoregulation of increasing circulation when nutrient value (oxygen & glucose) is low in blood is highly inefficient during shock. Availability of a nutrient to a cell is directly proportional to the blood flow & concentration of nutrient in the blood.

Glucose availability to a cell is proportional to the blood flow and blood glucose value

When blood glucose level falls a compensatory increase in blood flow can compensate for the decrease in blood glucose values. Coming to our discussion on seizures occurring during hypoglycemic attacks in newborns, we are not usually considering the perfusion part into the discussion. That may be the reason for the wide variation in manifestations of symptoms of hypoglycemia. For example, if blood sugar is low normal (e.g., 45 mg/dl) and perfusion is also borderline we can have a situation of relative low glucose supply to the neurons. This can result in seizures. In the same situation if perfusion was normal seizures would not have happened. Baby can have signs of sympathetic stimulation (tachycardia, sweating, jitteriness etc.) to compensate for a low blood sugar value. This sympathetic stimulation can increase perfusion.

Table: 10.1: Different scenarios of O2 & Glucose deficiency encountered by cells.

Different scenarios	Cellular effects	Interpretation
O2 supply normal with Blood hypoglycemia	Cells suffer hypoglycemia and ATP deficiency. Can compensate by increasing tissue perfusion.	There will be cellular hypoglycemia without increase in lactate.

Perfusion compromised (shock): (Here cellular availability of O2 & glucose low)	Glucose requirement increases 19 times, tissue level hypoglycemia occurs.	Compensation difficult unless shock improves
Oxygen low + hyperglycemia	Low O2 causes tissue level hypoglycemia which is Compensated to some extend by hyperglycemia.	Can compensate to some extend by increasing blood flow

Whenever cells undergo deficiency of glucose or oxygen, body tries to compensate through various mechanisms, the following are some of the mechanisms available.

1. Increasing blood flow by increasing heart rate and cardiac contractions, this is made possible by the release of counter regulatory hormones.
2. Increasing blood glucose levels through release of counter regulatory hormones (adrenaline, GH, renin – angiotensin, glucagon)
3. Giving extra oxygen helps in increasing dissolved oxygen content in the blood.
4. By decreasing tissue metabolism through cooling and by aggressively controlling seizures.

Chapter-11

How is a Uniform Brain Damage Produced in Severe CP & Acquired Microcephaly?

A baby born prematurely is at high risk of developing brain damage. The baby is at the mercy of the treating physician and nursing staff. The severity of insult can vary from very mild to severe injury. Severe extreme insult results in quadriplegic cerebral palsy and severe microcephaly. MRI of these unfortunate babies shows significant thinning of cerebral cortex, compensatory dilation of ventricles, severe PVL etc. Has anybody analyzed what has caused these damages at cellular level so extensively? Each and every cell (neurons, microglia, astrocytes oligodendrocytes etc.) in the brain is affected. What can cause such a nearly uniform damage? Such an insult is only possible with the shutting of supply, on which cells are highly dependent. There are only two substances on which cells are highly and continuously dependent, they are oxygen and glucose. Only inadequate perfusion (shock) can produce such a uniformly large deficiency where by both oxygen and glucose are in short supply. Severe asphyxia can also produce such a uniform injury where only oxygen supply is affected. Severe shock of short duration or mild shock (subtle shock) of long duration can produce same degree of insult. Both these (asphyxia & shock) can produce severe insult to tissues. Cerebral edema due to various causes like, encephalitis autoimmune encephalitis, IEM, severe continuous seizures, severe HIE, severe electrolyte abnormalities etc. can produce extensive cerebral destruction. A thrombosis or a hemorrhage in an arterial territory can produce injury restricted to that area. The following insults can produce uniform and widespread brain damage.

1. Severe oxygen supply disruption as in asphyxia
2. Severe shock (Terminal shock)
3. Uncompensated shock
4. Compensated shock
5. Subtle shock of long duration
6. Severe blood hypoglycemia
7. Severe cerebral edema due to various causes
8. Or any of the above combinations

As mentioned in the previous chapters, shock can produce severe insult through the mechanism of **Tissue level hypoglycemia**. Each and every cell undergo damage and result in severe microcephaly. For microcephaly to occur there should be global tissue destruction. A hemorrhage or a local arterial occlusion cannot produce such a uniform lesion. Next time when you see an acquired microcephaly child, think of an insult which had affected all cells. It is none other than a missed subtle shock, shock, asphyxia or a blood hypoglycemia.

Why was subtle shock not given much clinical importance till now?

From my observation, subtle shock, in fact, shock itself is not give its due respect or aggressiveness while treating. This may be due to the missing link of connecting shock with tissue damage. Tissue level hypoglycemia if proved at cellular level can act as a missing link connecting these two. The following are my points, why subtle shock was not given its due respect.

- One of the reasons is its difficulty in defining or measuring subtle shock. Subtle shock is not a single value or entity. There is a tendency to define everything in terms of absolute values. Subtle shock cannot be confined to such a frame. It has many variables which are observer dependent like Capillary refill time (CRT), appearance or color of the baby, degree of activity etc. There is also a tendency of sweeping things under the carpet which are difficult to define or measure.

- Exact normal NIBP values in a preterm or term babies are not fixed yet. There are wide variations and no absolute values. Don't know whether the obtained values are a result of compensation or not. If this is due to compensation then you can be sure that there is underlying shock which was masked by a normal BP. So sometimes compensatory signs may be missed. The list of signs of compensation are very vast and observer dependent.

- The degree of compensation is difficult to measure.

- There is a new tendency of moving away from clinical signs and symptoms to absolute definable values and investigations. At least some of the clinicians are challenging the reliability of CRT. It is a fact that CRT is a highly observer dependent variable, but in the clinical setting it still has some value.

- Modern medicine is giving less importance to clinical signs and symptoms. A baby looking not good is an intuition feeling (collective processing of many factors by brain compared with previous experiences) which is difficult to define verbally. When asked to define this intuition then you are in trouble.

- Subtle shock is a state of cellular deficiency of substrates, we are not able to co-relate this deficiency of cells with physical signs and symptoms. We have to discover more precise blood parameters which indicates this distress call from cells.

- For many symptoms like seizures, apnea, desaturations, lethargy exact molecular reasons for its occurrence are still unknown. Nobody tried to correlate it with subtle shock or shock. My conviction is that at least some of these are preventable if subtle shock is properly taken care of.

- If Prematurity is there then it takes most of the burden, everything is implied on prematurity. From experience, apnea is a nonevent (a rarity) for babies >30weeks unless there is shock or sepsis. Apnea of prematurity is a misnomer unless it is extremely premature (<28 weeks).

These are some of the reasons why subtle shock was never recognized as a clinical sign. Subtle shock was hidden from limelight and it silently destroyed our babies. Shock in any form should be taken seriously and stopping of an inotrope should not be our priority. Our priority should be to make sure all cells in the body are perfectly perfused. Slight over treatment of shock is not going to harm the baby. The contrary is silently devastating. Shock is a monster with unparalleled powers.

Chapter-12

Why is Theoretical Discussion Important for the Development of Science?

Science is an ever-expanding, never-ending experience. It is already fully manifest in the universe in its mightiest form. We humans are slowly rediscovering it one by one. We are slowly unravelling the science behind everything one by one at snail's pace. The creator has created everything with utmost perfection.

Wherever there is encouragement for free thinking and theoretical discussion new concepts get unravelled. For example, about the universe we know nothing, how it works, what are the theories surrounding black holes, how is life evolved, who is driving cellular functions, how gravity works, what is antimatter, dark matter, etc. all these are known to the universe and functioning perfectly. We are the one groping in the darkness.

For any science to grow first we have to encourage theoretical discussions, some people are genius who can use their imagination to arrive at far reaching conclusions. Later on, we can do experiments for proving it wright or wrong.

In the beginning of 20th century lots of theoretical sciences were flourishing like theoretical physics, theoretical chemistry, quantum mechanics, Einstein's theory of relativity etc. Several scientists were far ahead of time in thinking. Proving their theories took decades.

Table: 12.1: Time required to Prove Great Theories. (Power of theories)

Theories	Theorized	Discovered	Time required for discovery
Antimatter	1928	1932	4 years
Black holes	1916	1971	55 years
Higgs boson	1964	2012	48 years
Gravitational waves	1916	2015	99 years
Mendel work on inheritance of characters	1865	1900	35 years

The power of theories is great without which world would not have reached such great heights. Some people imagine things in their mind ahead of time with the available knowledge. I am mentioning this now because in the medical community there is a tendency of not accept anything without proof (Evidence-Based Medicine). A kind of over indulgence of "Evidence-Based Medicine" which has virtually killed theoretical discussions in medicine. No theory is accepted without proof. How can we bring proof even before picturing a theory? it is impossible. Evidence – based Medicine is absolutely needed but it should not eliminate theoretical discussions. First, when you are stuck with an idea, you theorise so many possibilities then you arrive at a conclusion and propose a hypothesis. This hypothesis is put in front of the scientific community for a wider discussion to see its relevance. Wider discussion brings about newer angles to the theory. This scrutiny by wiser people tests the theory whether it will stand or perish. Nowadays there are no wider discussions on new theories because theories are not coming into the limelight for discussion. This is because no publication is accepting publications based on theories, only studies are getting published (some of its relevance is a matter of debate). So, no wider discussions on new theories or hypothesis are happening because journal publication are forbidden for the majority as they need solid evidence for before publications. Wide variation from existing practice is never discussed.

Now a days majority of publications in major journals are useless comparisons and their comparisons are ridiculous. For example, I came across a publication in a major journal, lets us analyse it briefly.

Article name: The association of maternal weight on long-term neurodevelopmental outcome in premature infants (<29 weeks) at 18-24 months corrected age.

Objective: To determine the association of maternal pre-pregnancy body mass index (BMI) and neurodevelopmental impairment at 18-24 months corrected age in infants born <29 weeks gestation.

The conclusion is funny: Pre-pregnancy BMI was not associated with death or NDI in extremely preterm infants. Infants born to overweight mothers had higher odds of low language scores.

How on earth you do a study like this and arrive at such a conclusion, there are thousands and thousands of genetic, environmental variables and hormonal factors at play. The NICU stay for these babies cannot be standardized and only GOD knows the number of insults each baby have received. The two years of postnatal growth is highly variable from family to family. Family environment has a huge role to play in language development. The funny part is that there was no resistance for its publication, because these are the types of nonsense publications, we see in at least some journals.

Because of the need for solid evidences nobody is able to do ground breaking studies, all studies are not possible in humans. Can we encourage animal studies for fundamental research. Of course, before applying to patients, we need solid evidence. Before we do studies encourage open discussion on core concepts on which we are in darkness by involving experts. These kinds of discussions are not seen promoting in conferences or in journals.

Has too much Evidence – based Medicine killed scientific progress in medicine? There should be balance between **Evidence-based Medicine & Practice-based Evidence.**

References

1. Ganong's Review of medical physiology, 26th Ed, Gas transport between the lungs and the tissues. Publication; Mc Graw Hill – Lange medical book.

2. Granchi C, Bertini S, Macchia M, Minutolo F. Inhibitors of lactate dehydrogenase and their therapeutic potentials. Curr Med Chem. 2010;17 (7):672-97. (PubMed)(reference).

3. Peek CB, Levin Dc, Cedernaes J, et al. Circadian Clock interaction with HIE 1a Mediates oxygenic metabolism and anaerobic Glycolysis in skeletal muscle cell metabolism. 2017 Jan 10;25(1):86-92 (PMC free article) (PubMed) (reference list).

4. Basu SK, et al. Arch Dis Child fetal Neonatal Ed. 2017. PMID 27799322 Clinical trial. (Post hoc analysis of the Cool Cap Study).

5. Volpe, Neurology of the newborn, 5th Ed: page – 88.

6. Farmer SF, Harrison LM, et al. Plasticity of central motor pathways in children with hemiplegic cerebral palsy, neurology 41: 1501-1510, 1991.

7. Maegaki Y, Yamamoto T, et al. Plasticity of central motor and sensory pathways in a case of unilateral extensive cortical dysplasia: Neurology 45: 2255-2261,1995.

8. Uemastu J, Onu K et al. Development of corticospinal tract fibers and their plasticity. II. Neonatal unilateral cortical damage and subsequent development of the corticospinal tract in mice, Brain dev 18: 173 – 178, 1996.

9. Volpe Neurology of the newborn, 5th Ed: page 599-600.

10. Eda Cengiz, William V, Tamborlane, A tale of two compartments: Interstitial Versus Blood Glucose monitoring. Diabetes Technol Ther. 2009 Jun; 11 (Suppl 1): S-11–S-16. doi: 10.1089/dia.2009.0002

11. Finnemore A, Groves A. Physiology of the fetal and transitional circulation. Semin Fetal Neonatal Med. 2015 Aug; 20(4): 210-6. (PubMed).

12. Morton SU, Brodsky D. Fetal Physiology and transition to Extrauterine Life. Clin Perinatol. 2016 Sep; 43 (3): 395-407, (PubMed).

13. Kailey Remien; Sapan H, Majmundar Physiology, Fetal Circulation, National library of Medicine (NIH) April 26, 2023.

14. Rajeev Kumar Verma, Desislava Keller et al. Decreased oxygen saturation levels in neonates with TGA: impact on appearance of cerebral veins in susceptibility – weighted imaging. Sci Rep. 2017; 7: 15471. Published online 2017 Nov 13. doi: 10.1038/s41598-017-15591-3. PMCID PMC5684390/PMID: 29133891.

15. Sudeepta K Basu, Jason l Salemi, Alistair J Gunn, Jeffrey R Kaiser, Hyperglycemia in infants with HIE is associated with improved outcomes after therapeutic hypothermia: a post hoc analysis of the CoolCap study: PMID 27799322, Doi:10.1136/archdischild-2016-311385

16. Kim E Barret, Ganong's Review of Medical Physiology, 26th Ed 2029.

17. Erica A, Melkonian, Mark P. Schury. Biochemistry, Anaerobic Glycolysis, NCBI Bookshelf. NIH, Statpearl (internet) Treasue Island (FL): statPearls publishing; 2023 Jan.

18. Alberts B, Johnson A, Lewis J, et al. Molecular Biology of the cell. 4th Ed. New York Garland Science; 2002

19. YueMei Zhang and Bhagu R Bhavnani. Glutamate-induced apoptosis in neural cells is mediated via caspase-dependent and independent mechanism involving calpain and caspase-3 protease & apoptosis inducing factor (AIF), BMC neuroscience 2006; Published online 2006 Jun 15. Doi 10.1186/1471-2202-7-49

20. F J Walther et al. Am J Dis Child. 1990 Oct, Cardiovascular effects of caffeine therapy in preterm infants

21. Jing Zhao, Fernando Gonzalez, et al. Apnea of Prematurity: from cause to treatment. Eur J Pediatr. 2011; 170 (9): 1097-1105. Published online 2011 Feb 8. Doi: 10.1007/s00431-011-1409-6